Let Your Body Do the Work

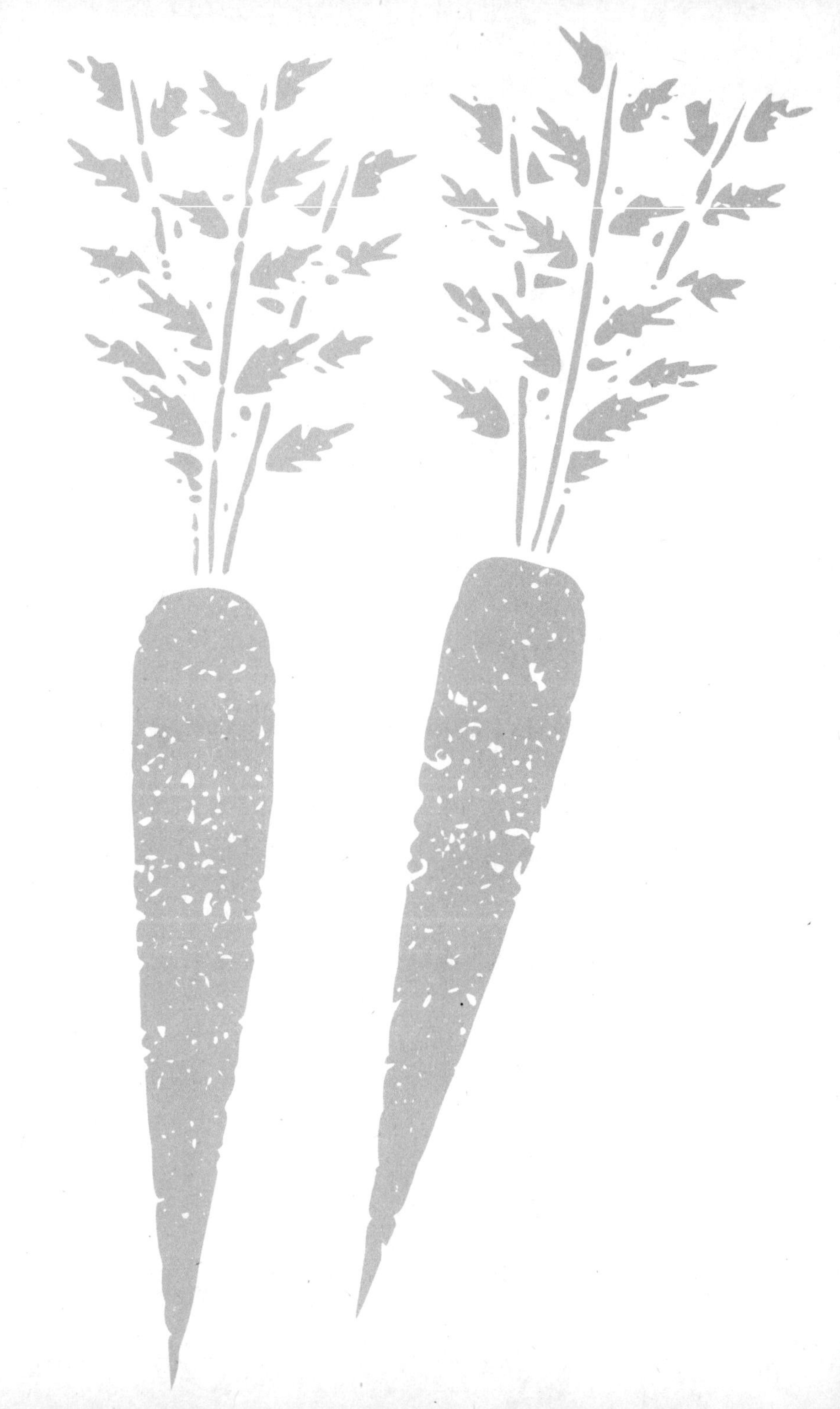

Let Your Body Do the Work

Activate Your Naturally Occurring GLP-1 Hormones for Healthy, Sustainable Weight Loss and Long-Term Health

ANETTE SAMS

translated by Paul Russell Garrett

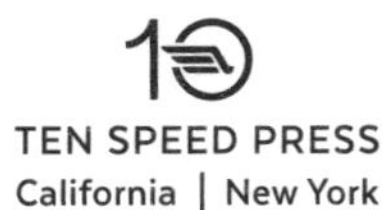

TEN SPEED PRESS
California | New York

TEN.SPEED PRESS
An imprint of the Crown Publishing Group
A division of Penguin Random House LLC
1745 Broadway
New York, NY 10019
tenspeed.com
penguinrandomhouse.com

A Ten Speed Press Trade Paperback Original

Originally published in Danish as *Kroppen kan selv: Aktivér dine naturlige vægttabshormoner* by Gyldendal Nonfiktion, Copenhagen, in 2024.

Illustrations by Maria Bramsen/Momgrafic
Art by Grunge farm produce set and Shutterstock.com/Northern Owl

Typeface(s): Bold Monday's Quinn Text, Linotype's Avenir Next Pro, and Linotype's Didot Pro

ISBN 979-8-217-27310-2
Ebook ISBN 979-8-217-27311-9

Editor: Thea Diklich-Newell | Production editor: Serena Wang
Designer: Aubrey Khan | Design manager: Andrea Lau
Production: Dan Myers | Compositor: North Market Street Graphics
Copy editor: Amy J. Schneider | Proofreaders: Diana Drew and Surina Jain
Publicist: Kristin Casemore | Marketer: Joey Lozada

Manufactured in the United States of America

1st Printing

The authorized representative in the EU for product safety and compliance is Penguin Random House Ireland, Morrison Chambers, 32 Nassau Street, Dublin D02 YH68, Ireland, https://eu-contact.penguin.ie.

Your body is capable
of more than you think,
and you are smarter
than you realize!

Contents

Foreword by Professor Jens Juul Holst

In recent years, research into the gut's role in health and disease has received considerable attention, particularly when it comes to the fascinating hormone GLP-1 (glucagon-like peptide-1). As we explore the complexity of the human metabolism more deeply, our understanding of the natural production of GLP-1 in the gut becomes increasingly important.

GLP-1 is more than simply a hormone and template for producing one of the world's leading medications. It is a central player in the body's intricate dance between energy balance, appetite regulation, and glucose metabolism. The production of GLP-1 in the gut's sensor cells reflects a remarkable mechanism that reacts to the presence of certain nutrients in the gut and adjusts accordingly to contribute to our overall metabolic health. But what is the best way to encourage these sensor cells to produce GLP-1?

This key question is what Anette Sams boldly investigates and explores in this book. *Let Your Body Do the Work* illustrates how to trigger natural GLP-1 production and offers insight into the factors affecting its release. By combining scientific research with practical knowledge, Anette seeks to encourage a deeper understanding of the gut's role in metabolic regulation.

When setting off on this journey through the body's digestive system and the science behind GLP-1, it is easy to become fascinated by the mechanisms at work, but the potential implications for health and lifestyle are even more important to consider. Anette's exploration is not simply an academic endeavor—it is a step toward understanding how we can use the power of our own biology to improve our lives.

The book also takes an in-depth look at how our modern diet, characterized by ultra-processed food and frequent meals, can prevent food from reaching areas of the gut where some of the body's most important natural weight-loss hormones are produced. Anette emphasizes the importance of choosing unprocessed foods that nourish not only us, but also our gut bacteria, which play a key role in our health. She describes how a diet rich in plant cells—in symbiosis with gut microbiota—ensures that nutrients and signals can be delivered to the cells controlling the production of weight-loss hormones such as GLP-1.

I am only too happy to encourage the reader to dive into this wonderful book, which unveils some of the mysteries surrounding GLP-1 and its impact on human health.

"Let your body do the work," says Anette Sams of our natural ability to produce GLP-1, which is something that has been proven through my own research, not least in connection with the effects of obesity surgery. Anette Sams's book is of value to anyone who would like to understand how their body works and how they can support its optimal functioning. Her enthusiasm for the subject shines through on every page, and her commitment to sharing this knowledge is admirable. I am confident that readers will find tremendous value in the insights and advice presented here.

Scientific communication is built on questions, hypotheses, and scientific disclaimers, while well-researched popular science must strive to posit answers for people to make use of. Few people can master the balancing act between the two, and Anette Sams is one of them.

She makes it relevant, interesting, and practical, while still maintaining the scientific disclaimers that keep the scientific path pure.

Anette is advocating for the everyday person, which is both commendable and respectable. I hope people will embrace the meaningful explanations, the fascinating story, and not least the solid dietary recommendations.

Enjoy!
Professor Jens Juul Holst

Jens Juul Holst is a professor at the Department of Biomedical Sciences at the University of Copenhagen. He is a pioneer in the discovery of GLP-1 and in describing its functions within the body, and has written hundreds of scientific articles on the topic. Jens Juul Holst is also the author of the book The Story of GLP-1.

Chapter 1

Meet your capable body

My country of Denmark as I knew it changed in December 2022. Only a few years earlier, the United States had debuted the medication that would take the world by storm, and now packs of the world's first plausible weight-loss medicine were flying off the shelves at pharmacies from Ringkøbing to Rønne. Wegovy, Novo Nordisk's brilliant replica of one of the body's natural weight-loss hormones, and the medication I'll refer to most here as it's the one I worked directly with, appeared like a rainbow on a rainy day. And for the way the world took to it, you'd believe that a pot of gold awaited those who could find the end of the rainbow.

In the story of Novo Nordisk and Wegovy,[*] the rainbow did in

---

[*] While there are multiple GLP-1 analog medications in the market, I will primarily be referring here to Wegovy (the medication I worked with) and Novo Nordisk, the creator of Wegovy and the company at which I worked for fifteen years. It's also important to note that Wegovy, and others such as Zepbound from Eli Lilly, are GLP-1 analog medications created for weight control, while other recognizable names such as Ozempic, also from Novo Nordisk, and Mounjaro, from Eli Lilly, are specifically

fact lead to gold. But for Wegovy users, the prize is a different story. Rather than a pot of cold cash awaiting them at the end of the rainbow, it's a dream finally realized. For millions of people around the world, their deepest wish appears to have been answered. With a click in the abdomen using a small pen, they are able to tame their constant hunger, which normally holds them captive, much like an unassailable dictator. At the same time, they're able to fulfill their desire to rid themselves of extra pounds around the waist, which despite restraint, constant deprivation, long plodding runs, and trips to the gym never quite seem to disappear for good.

The impact of Wegovy usage is tangible. Supermarkets report declining food sales and restaurants are serving smaller portions, while airlines spot an opportunity to save on fuel and improve their carbon footprint. People around the world face a slimmer—and perhaps healthier—future.

But with great discoveries come great dilemmas. This is also the case when looking at the success of Wegovy. Who needs the drug, and who is entitled to it? Who pays for it? There are those who steadfastly debate that obesity can be solved by riding your bike and practicing moderation in your eating choices; on the other side are those who can prove that appetite regulation and satiation are not simply a matter of willpower.

As a scientist, I'm not sure it's my place to posit an answer to any of those questions. But for me, there is no debate about sharing the knowledge and research on how to activate your

---

intended for management of type 2 diabetes. While the lifestyle interventions I discuss in this book can be beneficial for anyone, it's also important to speak with a doctor about what's best for you and your body.

naturally occurring GLP-1. It is up to you (and ideally your doctor) whether you want to use it. For my part, now that these medications are out in the world, I simply want to ensure that everyone can find the answers and education they need.

In addition to the ethical questions surrounding the use of Wegovy, the world's primary care physicians had to cope with the long line of people suddenly wanting the medication; elsewhere, second-party sellers popped up promising the same benefits with less regulation. The question raised here is perfectly banal: How can doctors and medical professionals ensure that treatment is carried out as the prescription demands—for Wegovy and other weight-loss medications to be used in combination with a healthy diet and exercise, as intended by its creators? In addition, who determines what the healthy diet that should accompany Wegovy consists of?

Wegovy gives rise to many questions, but no matter how much we wrestle with them, the medication continues to strengthen its presence around the world, and new generations of weight-loss medication are already on their way. But after decades researching in this space, I want people to understand that they have the tools to mimic the changes offered by these drugs at their fingertips, for a fraction of the price. It's time for everyone to learn about the fantastic and perfectly natural hormone underlying the astronomical success of these drugs—and it's created right in your own body.

The name of this hormone will tie your tongue in knots. Try it yourself: "glucagon-like peptide 1" . . . more commonly known as GLP-1. This is one of the hormones that balances your blood sugar, your appetite, and your weight. And the fantastic part is that your body can produce it on its own.

When it comes to your health, GLP-1 is a pack leader. When you eat good food that stimulates your body to produce the hormone, other hormones also join in, creating your own "health team." As the body continues to activate numerous other health switches, a positive feedback loop is created, laying a path to health, weight loss, and a body working in harmony. Because you can let your body do the work! That is, when you support it and get out of its way.

You probably think I'm now going to say that Wegovy is a pile of junk that should be chucked in the garbage in favor of the "natural" path to achieve a flat stomach. Nothing could be further from the truth. Wegovy is a brilliant quantum leap, and as a society, we have been in desperate need of a drug to break the obesity epidemic ravaging large parts of the world. But it is up to you and your doctor whether you choose the natural hormone, the artificially produced one, or both. My position is simply this: No one who seeks knowledge should be left without it.

This book is all about the body's natural weight-loss hormones, and it is for those who want to educate themselves and find the freedom to take charge of their own health. It's for those who believe in their capable body and know that health is never black and white. It's written in a scientist's voice, and from a scientist's perspective, because the information is the same whether you are reading this to kick-start your weight-loss journey, manage your type 2 diabetes, pursue the benefits of these popular weight-loss medications without the price tag and potential side effects, or simply educate yourself on a healthier way to live.

I am not writing a book about the hormone that inspired Novo Nordisk's talented experts for fun. I am doing it because I feel obligated to share this knowledge with you, and with the world. If you eat food, and if you want to learn a little more about what you can achieve when you let your body do the work, you will benefit from it.

Now, let's move quickly on to what so much of the hype around Wegovy centers on: weight.

Chapter 2

Definition of a public health crisis

Before tackling the body's built-in weight-loss hormones, you should understand a little more about the terms *obese, overweight, underweight,* and *healthy weight.* A lot of people bridle when confronted with these terms, but in order to have a fit and healthy body, it is important to grasp the fundamentals of these four labels.

But even before that, it is crucial to understand that a calorie (a unit of energy) outside the body does not translate 1:1 with a calorie inside the body. While some calories cost energy to absorb, other calories are absorbed free of charge. And while some calories are fully absorbed without activating any of the health benefits in your digestive system, you only gain access to others when they have triggered your digestive system and sparked a minor health revolution in your body.

In the coming pages, I will also explain why sugar is not simply sugar, that a weight-loss hormone administered by injection does not necessarily have the same effect as a weight-loss hormone produced in a specific part of the body, and that when it comes to both your internal and external health ecosystems, it is a matter of being in the right place at the right time with the right capabilities and the right partners—everything from friends and family to healthy gut bacteria.

Last but not least, I want to underline that no two people are exactly the same when it comes to food preferences, weight, energy levels, and the consequences of blood sugar swings. These are hard scientific facts that cannot be disputed. Regardless of diet, lifestyle, or exercise, everybody's ability to remove excess sugar from the blood, and the potential to influence that ability in a positive and negative direction, is going to be different. Since we are going to talk about both sides of the coin here, *insulin sensitivity* and *insulin resistance,* I want to be clear on this point.

But let's return to the term *obesity.* In my home country of Denmark, it is not considered a public health crisis, yet in other places in the world, including the United States and the UK, it is. In 1997, the World Health Organization (WHO) formally recognized obesity as a global epidemic, and the number of obese adults and children around the world has only increased since then. I am in no doubt as to what I believe, informed by decades of obesity research at Novo Nordisk: For some, obesity is a chronic illness requiring medication, but for the vast majority, obesity results from the fact that the human body cannot tolerate the lifestyles we have come to normalize, with diets of ultra-processed food and (in many cases) a lack of exercise, for a sustained period of time. I do not share this information to shame anyone, as I am well aware that food inequality is a real issue and access to education and resources are not available to all; my aim here is simply to provide science-backed findings for public use.

Fortunately, the body can be restabilized when a healthy biological interplay between digestion and energy storage is re-established.

WHEN DEFINITIONS DIFFER

Science works with fixed formulas to determine whether you are considered obese, overweight, at a healthy weight or underweight.

The prevailing definitions refer to the so-called body mass index (BMI). BMI is a measurement of your weight in relation to your height.

The formula for BMI is as follows:

$$BMI = \frac{\text{Your weight (kg)}}{\text{Your height (m) x Your height (m)}}$$

You can also easily google a BMI calculator to do the math for you.

According to BMI, you are at a healthy weight if the result of the formula is between 18.5 and 24.9. If your number is lower than that, it indicates you are underweight, and if it is higher, it indicates you are overweight. A BMI over 30 indicates obesity.

Already, we are faced with challenges regarding the definitions, because studies show that a large group of people with a BMI between 26 and 27 live longest. How can it be true both that those proven to live a long time are technically overweight, *and* that doctors and medical professionals warn against being overweight because it can be harmful to your health?

To answer that, we have to take a closer look at the definitions and acknowledge that variations between people are a given, which is why there is no single "optimal health category" to fit everyone into.

I know a lot of people who exercise intensely and persistently to build muscle mass. They may have a BMI of around 30, made up mostly of muscle. On the other hand, I know other people with a BMI of 22 for whom the bulk of their weight is concentrated around the waist—precisely where we do not want it to be.

This is why it is neither appropriate nor suitable to use BMI as the sole indicator of health. Instead, it should be used as a guideline, in combination with a dose of common sense and an assessment of whether your fat deposits sit around your waist (also known as "unhealthy fat") or on your buttocks and thighs and generally evenly distributed across the body in the form of insulation (also known as "healthy fat"). Take this scientist's word for it—people in the overweight BMI category who are physically active are healthier than people who are physically inactive in the healthy body weight category.

If you choose to look beyond BMI, your waist measurement can place you in a new health category. Some recommendations suggest your waist should be less than half of your height. If you are 5-foot-3 (160 cm), your healthy waist measurement should be below 31½ inches (80 cm), and if you are 5-foot-10 (180 cm), it should be below 35 inches (90 cm).

A third method you can use to place yourself in a category is to use a smart scale that measures your body fat, the amount of fat in the stomach region, muscle mass, bone density, resting calorie consumption, and your biological age. If you've set yourself a health goal, it can be exciting and uplifting to follow the changes in the numbers on the scale. But these results can vary, depending on a number of factors, so setting yourself up in comparison to others based on these metrics can be hit-or-miss. For example, I can reveal that my biological age varies between twenty-five and fifty, while my actual birth certificate reveals that I was born in 1971.

With all that said, by all means calculate your BMI, measure the circumference of your waist, and use every health calculator available, if it makes you happy. But promise that you'll remember to stay focused on the best health calculator of them all—how you feel in both mind and body. These are health indicators that no formula or electronic gadget can measure.

In other words, I'd like to set your mind at ease. I give you permission to free yourself from the weight of norms, self-reproach, and unrealistic beauty ideals, and allow yourself to find independence and self-confidence when it comes to your health. This is one of the reasons you will not find a weight-loss plan in the following pages. Instead, you will find educational materials and a blueprint for an intuitive, supportive relationship to your body that gives you the freedom to be healthy and confident.

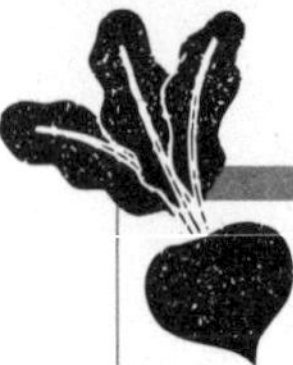

HOW DO YOU SEE YOURSELF?

When you are confronted with a significant change in your health, it's a good idea to look at yourself and your body.

- Are you overweight? Are you a healthy weight or do you weigh too little?

- Are your fat deposits around the belly or more evenly distributed?

- Is your weight a health concern?

- Is your weight a cosmetic concern?

- Would you like to lose weight?

- How much would you like to lose?

Once you have answered these, the million-dollar question is: Why do you want to lose weight? The answer to that is key to your motivation to lose weight, and once that is established, you'll be in a better position to assess how much you'd like to invest in your goal and how much you are willing to sacrifice to achieve it. That is, if you choose to see it as a sacrifice—because only you can answer that. But there's a really good chance that what you consider a sacrifice today will soon be something you're only too happy to give up.

But back to the key to your desire to lose weight. Once that is established, you should ask yourself three further questions to help you on your way.

- On a scale of one to ten, how important is losing weight to you?

- Imagine you've achieved your desired weight. What would that mean for your mood, your daily routine, and your enjoyment of life?

- What would it mean if once and for all you said to yourself: I weigh what I weigh, but starting today, I'd like to understand my body a little better and see what it feels like if I work with it and not against it?

FACTORS CONTRIBUTING
TO BECOMING OVERWEIGHT

In recent years, so much has been written about how we don't know why so many people become overweight, and how we have no idea how to achieve lasting weight loss.

I disagree with these two assertions. There are ways people become overweight, and there are ways people can get out of being overweight. The fact is, we rarely ask the right questions to solve these dilemmas. Research on people who have been able to sustain lasting weight loss is insufficient. The same goes for research on individuals who almost never gain weight.

Some people become overweight from eating too much. Or from eating the wrong things. Other people become overweight because they do not include enough physical activity in their lives, while some people become overweight from not eating enough—by this, I don't necessarily mean they're not eating enough calories, but that they're not eating enough of the foods that can activate the main biological health switches in the body, which the "wrong" food never reaches.

Further to that, I want to mention the phenomenon known as *insulin resistance*. Insulin resistance can make people feel as though they don't have enough energy, even when they have consumed plenty of calories, potentially leading them to eat even more to try to attain that energy they were seeking. In this situation, the energy (calories from food) one has consumed floats around in the blood instead of settling in the right place, where it can be turned into energy by your body. In other words, it is not in the right place at the right time.

So here comes the first and most important message in this book: Your food should provide you with nutrients and energy *and* contribute to numerous vital mechanisms that support your long-term health.

Along with this message, I want to acknowledge the phenomenon known as *biological variation* among individuals. What is good for you and for yours is not necessarily good for me and mine, and what doesn't work on the average person might work on you. One size does not fit all. Chew on that for a moment. It is not so different from life in general—everyone knows you can take two completely different routes to reach the same result, and that the same path does not necessarily lead to the same result for different people.

By educating yourself about the body's weight-loss hormones, you're equipping yourself with the best tools—the best compass—to find the path leading you to a healthy body. There is so much noise in the health and wellness space; now is a good time to focus on yourself alone and accept that your path may not be relevant to others, just as their path may not lead you to your goal.

Which is why, when it comes to your personal health, you can only be responsible for yourself. Likewise, other people's health is a matter for them. I hope that you will use this book to kickstart your own journey. Beyond that, you can use your new knowledge to set a good example and inspire the people you care about.

Chapter 3

The body's biological weight-loss medication

The weight-loss medication Wegovy is not the only ground-breaking medicine from Novo Nordisk, which on an almost daily basis makes headlines around the world. Ozempic, a medicine for type 2 diabetes, entered the market before Wegovy. One thing the two medicines have in common is that they contain the medication semaglutide, which brilliantly mimics the effect of GLP-1, the body's own naturally occurring gut hormone.

Semaglutide regulates blood sugar and appetite, affects food preferences, and—along with exercise and a low-calorie diet—can lead to significant weight loss. It also reduces the risk of car-diovascular disease, kidney disease, and dementia, among other things, which are higher in people with diabetes who are also overweight.

As the fantastic results continue to pour in, semaglutide is now something requested by the average person. Doctors tell me the two medications have changed their everyday experiences at their practice. All of a sudden, doctors are dealing with patients they do not normally hear from, who describe lifelong battles with weight, in the hopes of being prescribed Wegovy. And doctors see aggressive patients demanding a prescription because they believe they're entitled to the same help as their neighbor.

Let's conduct a little thought experiment. Imagine you ask your doctor for help overcoming your excess weight. Your doctor suggests discussing whether you will benefit more from the medication, or whether you should first find out together if your body's natural weight-loss hormones can have a significant impact. How would you respond? Would you reject your doctor's suggestion straightaway? Or would you choose to activate your body's natural hormones?

There is no right or wrong answer here, because no matter what you choose, the most important thing is the thought process around your decision. From my perspective, keeping an open mind as you discuss the choice between Wegovy and lifestyle adjustments, and the ensuing activation of the body's natural hormones such as GLP-1, can help patient and doctor have conversations where blame and shame do not dominate and arrive at a customized plan that works in the patient's best interests.

THE MAGIC HORMONE

Briefly, a hormone is a biological signaling molecule that functions as a messenger in the body. Insulin, for example, is a hormone that regulates your blood sugar, while the sex hormones—estrogen and testosterone—are crucial for the development of sex characteristics.

Hormones are produced in different glands and organs around the body, and they are transported via the body's personal highways—the arteries and veins. When hormones reach their destination, they carry out the exact job they are designed to perform. Basically, it's like taking the train to work, and if there are no delays on the tracks, you arrive on time to carry out your daily tasks. The only difference is that you return home at the end of the workday and leave again the following morning. Hormones, however, do not return home. Once they have completed their task, they are broken down into their basic components and excreted or repurposed into other vital substances in your body.

Let's look at the GLP-1 hormone, a so-called gut hormone formed in the cells of your digestive system. The entire digestive system is composed of your mouth, your stomach, your duodenum, your small intestine, and your large intestine. It is in these different spaces that the digestive processes occur. Add to that the two conveyor belts—the esophagus, which transports food from the mouth to the stomach, and the rectum, which transports food remnants out of your system and into the toilet—and you've got the full picture.

But the basics of the digestive system alone aren't enough to turn food into energy and the vital biological processes that secure long-term health. In each space, digestive assistance is provided by either the body's glands, which deliver acid, enzymes, and bile salts, for example, or from important microorganisms that reside in the digestive system, where they live in synergy with you and your health.

But let's pause there for a moment, because you have to remember these microorganisms. They are your most important allies, so we'll come back to them.

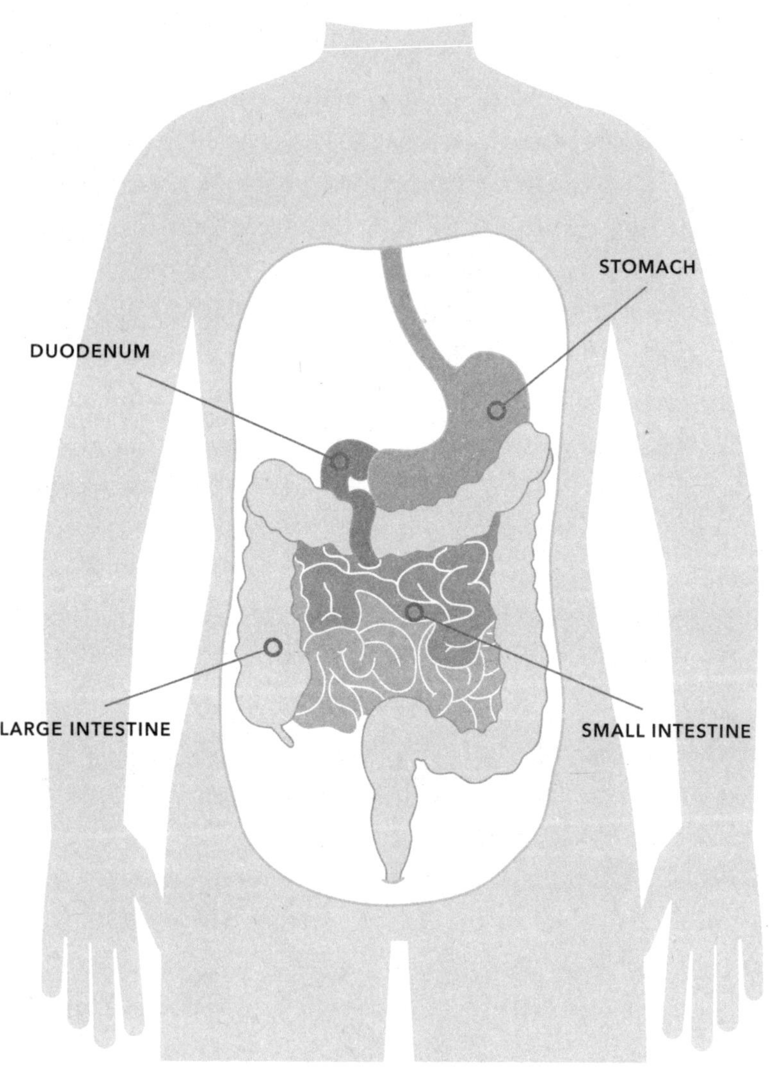
STOMACH
DUODENUM
LARGE INTESTINE
SMALL INTESTINE

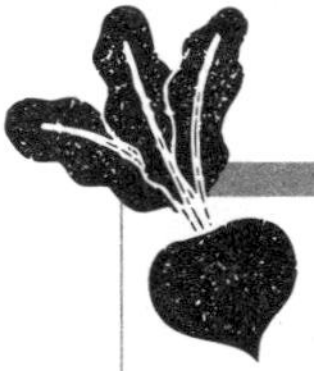

THE ANATOMY OF DIGESTION

As food travels down your esophagus and into your twenty-six-foot (8 m) digestive system, several processes occur, which you can neither see nor consciously control . . . until it is time to flush what remains down the toilet. There are a number of digestive processes.

PHYSICAL PROCESSES consist of, among other things, pulverization through chewing, suspension and dissolution of the chewed food in the body's digestive fluids, churning through rhythmic contractions of the gut, and the formation of small "fat shuttles," which wrap fat inside a bubble so it can be transported from the gut and into the lymph and the bloodstream.

CHEMICAL PROCESSES include the decomposition of food when it comes in contact with stomach acid, while the *enzymatic processes* include the breakdown of starch (polysaccharides) into sugar (monosaccharides), and the breakdown of proteins into amino acids.

The effort required of your body during digestion is extensive, before monosaccharides, amino acids, and fats can be funneled away from the digestive system and into the bloodstream, where they are distributed in the body.

Let's take a quick trip through the digestive system, starting from the top—to be more precise, the mouth, where the teeth are designed to bring about the initial "demolitions." This is where you chew the food to break it into smaller pieces, sampling it with your taste buds and mixing it all with enzymes and water from your saliva.

The food moves quickly down through the esophagus to the stomach, where it is combined with acid, which among other things aids digestion and kills unwanted bacteria.

In the duodenum, your pancreas neutralizes the stomach acids, after which enzymes are added. If the enzymes manage to get hold of the essential nutrients (carbohydrates, fat, and protein), this is where the breakdown of nutrients into smaller molecules—sugar, amino acids, and fatty acids—begins. But once the molecules of the essential nutrients are broken down into smaller units, the body, via the intestinal mucosa's barrier cells, can transport the nutrients into the bloodstream, where they are distributed to the entire body to be used as energy, signaling molecules, or building blocks.

With the smaller nutrients gone, the remaining food passes farther down into the small intestine with the aid of rhythmic contractions of the intestines. Movement and digestion take place simultaneously, so believe me when I say that your digestive system really can multitask!

The processes within your intestines all happen in a particular order. Think of the digestive system as a railway station, with different trains passing through it all day. To ensure a smooth departure on the correct train, the digestive system monitors how many and which passengers are traveling to the next destination. All to ensure that everything is where it should be when the train and all the passengers arrive at the next stop on their journey. In other words:

- The digestive system digests food (breaks it into smaller units that can be transported into the bloodstream).

- The digestive system monitors digestion like a control tower (how many nutrients, flavor compounds, and so on, travel into the bloodstream).

- The digestive system prepares the body for what is coming (sends signals to the body so everything admitted into the bloodstream ends up in the right place).

- The digestive system prepares for the arrival of the next meal (increases or decreases appetite).

- The digestive system prepares the immune system for what is coming (so the immune system can combat, for example, an unwanted invasion of dangerous bacteria).

This monitoring, aided by the gut's sensor cells and signals from the gut hormones that emanate from the sensor cells, is the most fascinating and crucial point.

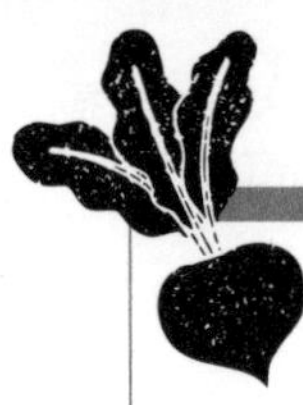

THE UNEXPECTED LESSON OF BARIATRIC SURGERY

It is a well-known fact that people get fuller faster and eat less if the size of their stomach is surgically reduced. So it is not surprising that various surgical interventions on the stomach and the duodenum have a positive effect on people experiencing obesity. But scientists also came across some unexpected findings from these operations when they studied their effects on the GLP-1 hormone. To understand why, it's important to know that this surgery removes the lower part of the stomach as well as the duodenum, meaning that digested food "jumps" to the intestines more quickly from the stomach.

Three surprising observations came out of long-term studies of the effects of this type of surgery:

- Medical science did not initially register that the absorption of nutrients and calories was reduced when both the stomach and the duodenum were surgically altered.

- Researchers have measured far more GLP-1 in the blood of people who have had the operation compared to those who either ate the same food or absorbed exactly the same nutrients but didn't undergo the surgery.

- People who experienced obesity with type 2 diabetes saw drastic, immediate effects in their blood sugar levels directly following the surgery, even before they lost weight, meaning that the operation—regardless of weight—must stabilize high blood sugar, which is difficult to curb in people with diabetes.

Although the analyzed operations had the expected result, namely severe weight loss, the implications for the body's own weight-loss hormone, GLP-1, and the effect that GLP-1 has on the body's blood sugar must also be studied.

Let me reiterate the importance of these takeaways for our conversation surrounding the GLP-1 hormone:

The weight loss triggered by bariatric surgery is not only the result of the person consuming fewer calories. It is also due in large part to the fact that the meals encounter a smaller part of the digestive system (the stomach and the upper part of the gut are bypassed) following the operation. With the upper portion of the digestive system out of play, more undigested food reaches the later sections of the digestive system, meaning that food reaches the sensor cells that produce GLP-1 in a less-digested state than they do without the surgery. The takeaway is clear: Less-digested food triggers greater production of GLP-1 within the further sections of the intestines. But it does not stop there. This surgery leads to the production of a series of other hormones, which accompany GLP-1 from the gut's sensor cells. This will all be of note when we discuss the importance of the structure of food, specifically of foods that take longer to digest in the system, and how these can trigger your naturally occurring GLP-1 hormones.

THE ALL-IMPORTANT SENSOR CELLS

For the GLP-1 hormone, the millions of barrier cells separating your digestive system from the rest of your body are of particular interest. The barrier cells are densely packed on the inside of the gut, where with a firm hand and great precision they control what gets transferred into the blood and what continues down the gut for further digestion.

In the duodenum, specific barrier cells have an extra responsibility: While forming a barrier between the contents of the gut and the rest of your body, they also act as sensor cells and register what you have eaten. The barrier cells, which are simultaneously sensor cells, note the various nutrients from the food, and they accompany the absorption of nutrients with hormones that guide the nutrients to the right places in the body. One of these specialized sensor cells is called the *L-cell*.

This sensor cell secretes the weight-loss hormone GLP-1 and several other hormones. For that reason, sensor cells have been the subject of attention from some of the world's most accomplished researchers for decades. Why? Because GLP-1 and the other hormones that the sensor cells have tucked away have on several occasions turned our understanding of digestion and weight regulation on its head.

The hallmark of these great discoveries in the body is no different than other great discoveries: Clever people with an interest in a particular subject listen and speak to other clever people who are interested in something altogether different. Dialogue, disagreement, and mutual curiosity ensure that everyone becomes more knowledgeable. In the end, you agree upon a new theory. The new theory (later proven) posited that in the digestive system, different types of sensor cells are distributed in a particular pattern. We also learned that bypassing sections of the digestive system can make other parts of the digestive system produce much more GLP-1 than normal. It is simply a matter of reaching the sensor cells situated far down inside the intestines.

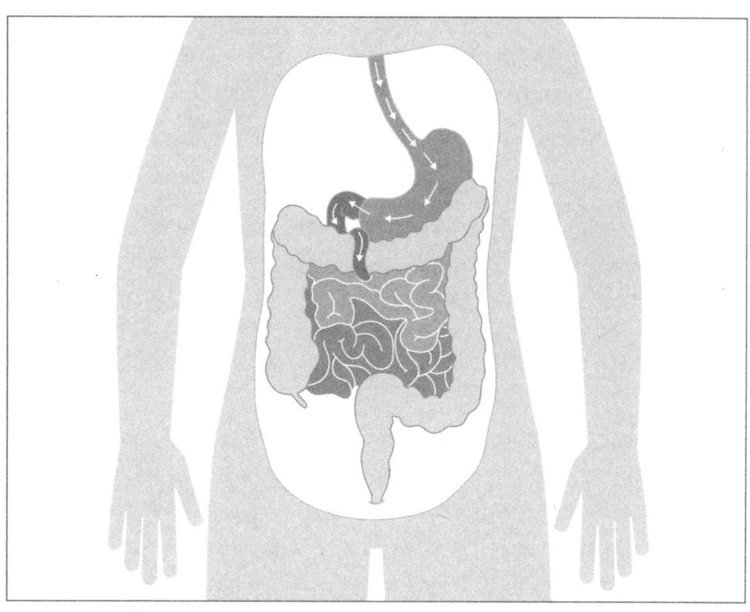

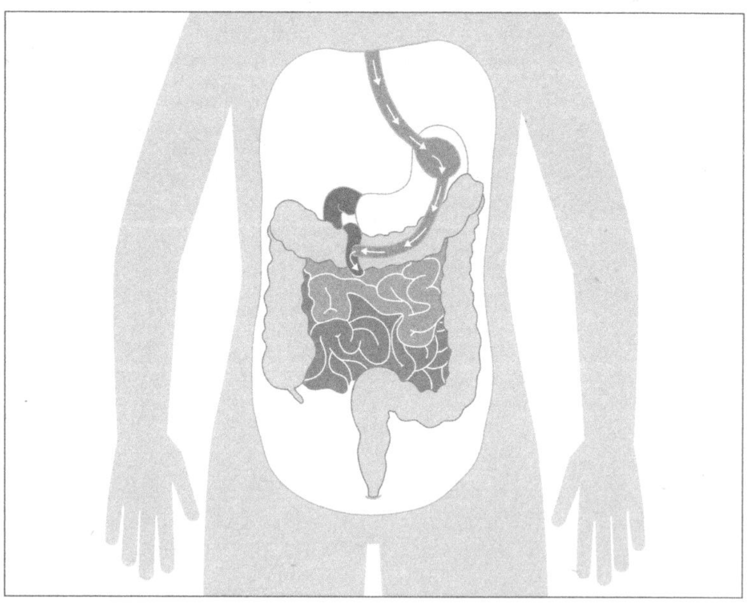

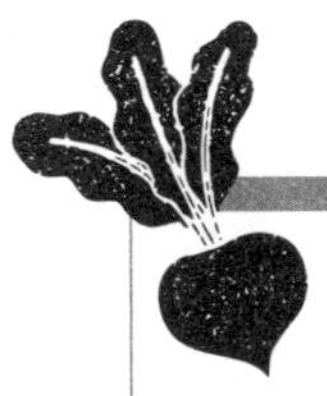

THE DIGESTIVE SYSTEM—
NATURAL AND RECONSTRUCTED

In your digestive system, food works its way through the stomach and out the duodenum, where it continues through the small intestine and the large intestine, before the digested food and a series of bacterial remnants end up in the toilet.

Years ago, researchers discovered that an obesity operation, which created a direct shortcut between a much smaller stomach and the small intestine, meant that the patient's type 2 diabetes symptoms quickly disappeared. For months and years afterward, the person would lose significant weight—which was precisely the aim of the operation. But the weight loss was much greater than medical science had anticipated. This wasn't a question of a simple correlation between food consumption and weight. This observation was central to the discovery of the all-important weight-loss hormones, and it turned out that more unprocessed food in the small intestine meant the production of more weight-loss hormones, which again led to unexpected weight loss and stable blood sugar.

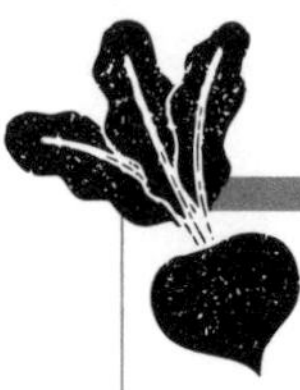

THE L-CELLS—
YOUR CAPABLE SENSOR CELLS

An L-cell is a barrier cell in your intestines that has an extra area of responsibility. In addition to forming barriers between the contents of the gut and the rest of your body, it is equipped with sensors that detect and respond to what you have eaten.

One of the responses is to dispatch a dose of hormones that boosts your ability to remove sugar from the bloodstream and reduces your appetite. The most well-known hormone is GLP-1, but the L-cell is also well-stocked in PYY (polypeptide Y), which, among other things, regulates your sugar cravings, and GLP-2 (glucagon-like peptide-2), which boosts the barrier function of your gut.

L-cells and other barrier cells with sensory functions and the ability to produce hormones are also known as *enteroendocrine cells*. Directly translated, this means intestinal cells that can produce hormones. These cells play an important role in the digestive system, and they are more and more densely situated the farther down you go in the twenty-six-foot-long digestive system.

The L-cells are the sensor cells you ideally want to activate with your undigested food. When these cells sense nutrients in the gut attaching themselves to the taste receptors on their surfaces, they produce and distribute the weight-loss hormone GLP-1. The taste receptors—or the taste sensors—carry the same name as their counterparts in the mouth. But whereas taste receptors in the mouth are stimulated by molecules from your food, and the composition of the food determines whether you like a certain food, the taste receptors in the L-cells do not determine whether you like certain foods.

Instead, they determine how much GLP-1 needs to accompany your food. The L-cells, as mentioned, are situated between the barrier cells in the gut along the entire intestinal system—from the duodenum to the rectum. But the farther you travel into the small intestine, the more densely these highly GLP-1-producing gut cells are clustered. This essential knowledge may make you change your mindset when it comes to food.

It is one thing whether you consume the nutrients—fat, proteins, carbohydrates, vitamins, and minerals—you need. It is another thing altogether whether those nutrients reach the large fields of L-cells farther down the digestive system, or whether they reach only the few and scattered sensor cells in the duodenum and the upper part of the small intestine. Herein lies the problem—if the nutrients reach only the upper sensor cells and are absorbed only in the upper part of the gut, a large wave of nutrients will hit the bloodstream like a tsunami, which is why the hormones intended to guide the nutrients into position and regulate how much nutrition is needed simply can't keep up.

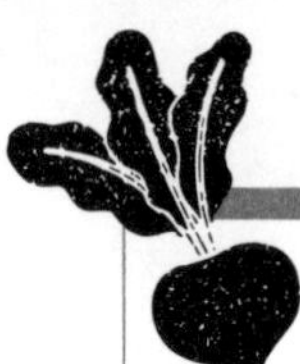

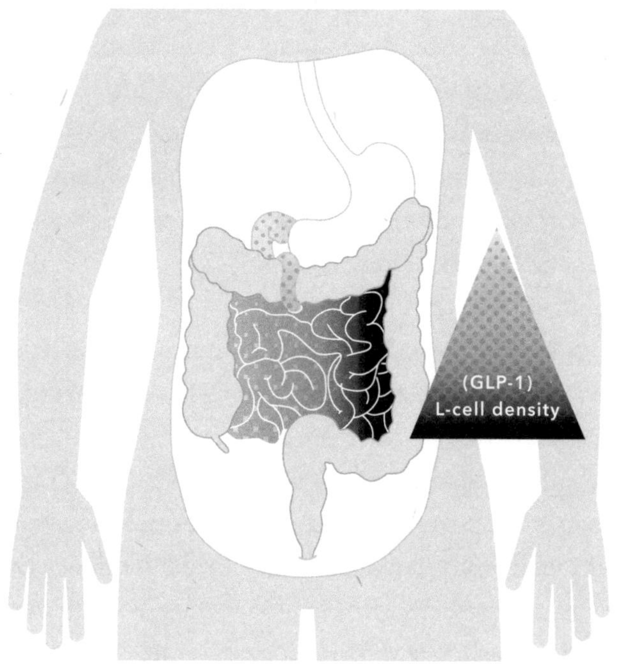

THE SENSOR CELLS IN DIFFERENT AREAS

The farther down we go in the small intestine, the more densely packed the L-cells, which produce GLP-1 to regulate your appetite and help stabilize your blood sugar, are. And that is not all. GLP-1 is not the only health facilitator released by these sensor cells. As well as GLP-1, hormones like GLP-2, GIP (gastric inhibitory polypeptide), and PYY help strengthen your body's own prevent-and-treat healthcare system.

The question now is this: If you do not want—or are not eligible—to have most of your stomach and duodenum removed, then what is the best way to ensure that your L-cells receive the good, GLP-1-supporting nutrients? Backed by science, the solution is right in front of you.

- Eat unprocessed foods.

- Vary your diet—preferably with lots of vegetables.

- Aim for a combination of cooked and raw produce.

Can you picture it? If you eat both raw and cooked vegetables (which require different degrees of digestion), nutrients from the food will be absorbed along the entire length of the gut—all twenty-six feet of it. And because the food reaches the final feet of the intestine, you'll also feed the areas of your digestive system where you have the most sensor cells capable of producing GLP-1.

So activating your body's natural weight-loss hormones is actually quite simple. What it all boils down to is this: Eat an unprocessed, vegetable-rich diet—that's it! But stick with me, because I'm going to continue to provide you with the tools to do this right.

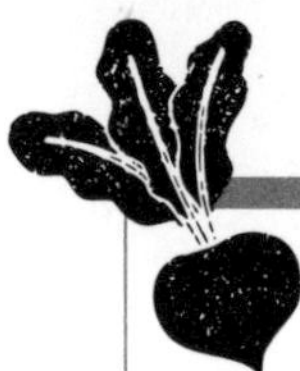

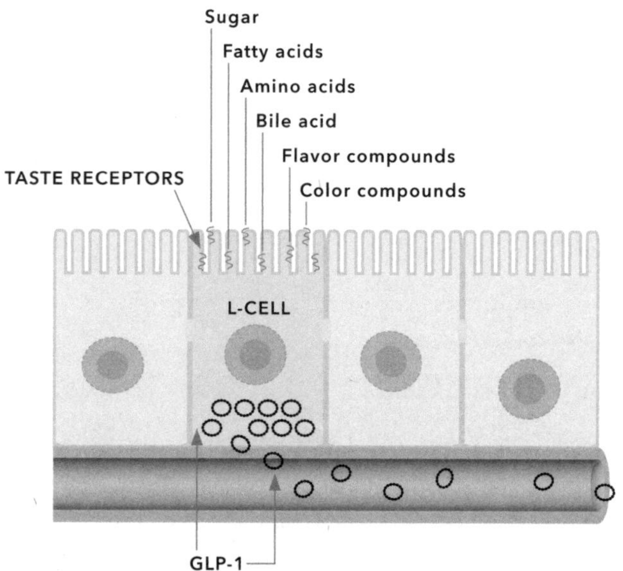

YOUR FRIENDLY GUT CELLS

Arranged in tidy rows throughout the digestive system are barrier cells and sensor cells, which together we call *epithelial cells*. Most epithelial cells are barrier cells that transport nutrients from the digestive tract into the bloodstream.

The farther down we go in the twenty-six-foot-long digestive system, the more densely packed we find the kind of epithelial cells that release GLP-1, namely, the L-cells.

On the surface of the L-cells are various taste receptors. The taste receptors are activated by nutrients (from fat, carbohydrates, and protein) and flavor and color compounds (for example, plant chemicals) from your food. The receptors are also activated by the bile acid from your digestive system and a wide range of other substances created by the millions of different microorganisms living in your gut, which are primarily responsible for the digestion of plant-based foods. When the taste receptors on the surface of the L-cells are activated, the cells receive a signal to release a portion of GLP-1 molecules.

And there you have it! This activation of weight-loss hormones is something you can benefit from—regardless of how much you weigh—because the bodily effects of GLP-1 are far-reaching and significant.

Overall, GLP-1 molecules can do one of four things in your body. I'll mention them here and we'll explore more later on:

- They can act locally on nearby cells via the GLP-1 receptors.

- They can activate receptors and produce nerve signals affecting your appetite and sense of satisfaction and satiety, among other things.

- They can permeate into the bloodstream, where they are transported to GLP-1 receptors around the entire body.

- They can—either before or after they have started to do their work—be degraded, so they can no longer function. After the degradation, GLP-1's component parts are recycled by the body.

Chapter 4

How your body produces its own natural weight-loss hormone

Before we look at what foods are guaranteed to take long enough to digest that they are sure to deliver nutrients to the L-cells, you should know that there are several ways to *boost* your production of GLP-1.

Let's start with the muscles. When you use your muscles, for example when you go for a run, lift weights at the gym, or take a horseback ride in the woods—anything that makes the lactic acid in your muscles burn a little—your muscles require more blood. Blood ensures that your muscles get sufficient oxygen while also returning waste products to the kidneys to be excreted or to the liver to be recycled. At the same time, neurotransmitters are released from the many different nerves winding around the small arteries in and around the working muscles. And this is where it gets interesting, because in addition to enlarging local blood vessels, neurotransmitters can also stimulate the gut's L-cells into circulating GLP-1—but only if the neurotransmitters make it all the way down to the L-cells before the body has either broken them down or disposed of them.

When it comes to the release of GLP-1, one of the most exciting neurotransmitters is CGRP. Becoming an expert on CGRP is not required, far from it—you don't even need to know what the abbreviation stands for. All you need to know is that CGRP functions as your body's own little SOS signal, which, if an area of the body lacks oxygen, rushes out of the nerve endings and increases blood flow exactly where the oxygen shortage is, and nowhere else.

Since the start of the millennium, I've been infatuated with CGRP. CGRP is a peptide—an organic compound made up of thirty-seven amino acids conveying signals between cells and regulating various biological processes. I am now researching whether it is possible to create a CGRP medication that can provide the body with reliable assistance, for example, when it lacks oxygen in the heart because of severe blood clots. Forgive me for this digression—but it illustrates how the body has the most unbelievable rescue boats at its disposal when we get into deep water.

Back to the working muscles. Exercise and neurotransmitters, which the central nervous system uses to regulate blood supply—along with the undigested food that reaches deep inside the gut—play a part in how much GLP-1 is produced by your body. Here it might be reasonable to think that you should just exercise a lot and eat a lot. Unfortunately, it's not that simple. Biology is rarely that simple. Gut hormones are no exception, and a full stomach is particularly guilty of producing hormones that reduce—practically prevent—the formation of GLP-1 in the upper L-cells. But we can find a way around that!

To summarize: Get regular exercise, take breaks between meals (meaning periods with an empty stomach or fasting for a few hours, something I will return to), and eat lots of vegetables, which are perfect for transporting nutrients farther down the gut. This is the way forward if you want to try to produce as many natural weight-loss hormones as possible.

Chapter 5

What can you choose to eat?

Earlier I wrote that L-cells have an abundance of taste receptors on their surface. "Taste receptors" may sound a little off-putting, but fortunately you cannot taste what is moving around inside your gut. This is despite the fact that the taste receptors in your intestines are almost indistinguishable from the ones in your mouth, even though they do something very different. But what exactly are these taste receptors?

Let's start in the mouth. The densely packed taste receptors in your taste buds note when you perceive sweet, sour, salty, bitter, and umami. These five flavors are called *basic tastes*—a unique taste that can't be formed by combining other tastes. The basic tastes are more than flavor experiences. Each is a kind of direct line to the body, carrying information about the content of the food.

When the five basic tastes stimulate receptors in your taste buds, the receptors give you a sensory experience of "yum!" or "yuck!"—or other more subtle and complex taste experiences in between. All because the receptors emit signals about the basic tastes through your nervous system, allowing you to experience that particular taste.

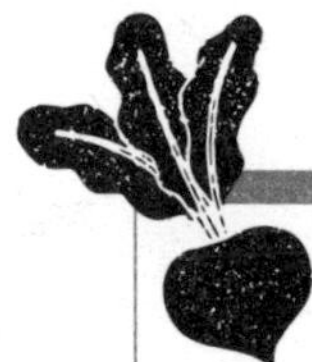

SOUR

There is acid present in the food.
This could be a sign of unripe or tainted food.

SWEET

Sweetness indicates there is sugar in the food,
meaning the food contains lots of energy.

SALTY

If food tastes salty, the body knows the
food contains salts, which are important
for the functioning of the body.

BITTER

The food could be poisonous.

UMAMI

This taste signals that the food is rich in protein.

The function of the taste receptors in the gut is something altogether different. When you stimulate these taste receptors, you do not get a conscious sensory experience; on the contrary, a number of processes occur without you realizing it. This stimulation in the gut ensures, among other things, that packages of GLP-1 molecules are released into the body, and that you send messages via the nervous system, which lies under the gut's barrier cells. Although you do not exclaim, "Aha! Now the taste receptors in my gut are being stimulated," a lot of new research suggests that this stimulation still satisfies you and, among other things, reduces your cravings for *superstimuli* such as the food industry's magic concoction of sweet, salty, and fatty contained in ultra-processed food (which we will critique a little later).

Interestingly, research also shows that nearly all the food you consume can release substances that attach themselves to the L-cells. That goes for flavor compounds and for the essential nutrients: fat, protein, and carbohydrates. This is why I can't give you an Instagrammable recipe for how to build your meals based solely on nutrients and flavor compounds. There are simply so many different compounds in foods from all over the world—vegetables in particular—that can activate taste receptors.

For example:

Short-chain fatty acids, which are formed by microorganisms when they break down fiber from the walls of the plant cells during digestion in the large and small intestines.

Sugar, which is found in plant cells or is formed when the starch in vegetables is broken down by you and your gut microbes.

Various amino acids, which come from the breakdown of protein in your food—or are formed by microorganisms in your digestive system.

Plant chemicals, which are also called *phytochemicals* and include flavor and color compounds, as well as antioxidants found in our vegetables. They can also be breakdown products that are formed by your gut microbes.

Does that sound complicated? Maybe this will make it simpler: A vegetable contains thousands of plant cells. All plant cells are wrapped in fiber, which you and your body can't break down without assistance. This is absolutely brilliant, because the plant has a fiber envelope surrounding all of its nutrients and flavor and color compounds, ensuring that the myriad of components in the plant cell are transported to the taste receptors of the L-cells far down in the digestive system.

But how do we get all these substances to reach the taste receptors on the surface of the L-cells and how do we access GLP-1? This is where we are given a helping hand.

THE GHOST OF THE MEAT-COATED SKELETON

A few years ago, I came across a funny quote on the internet. It goes like this:

You are a ghost driving a meat-coated skeleton made from stardust, riding a rock, hurtling through space.

The quote is amusing because it is almost true. Maybe it should read like this instead:

You are a ghost driving a meat-coated skeleton made from stardust, riding a rock, hurtling through space, along with millions of microorganisms.

Because living in every single cubic centimeter of your gut are thousands of microorganisms, which, in symbiosis with your body, ensure that you live a healthy life. Many of the microorganisms do not even have a name, and they live off the fiber the plant cells are wrapped in. So the farther down the gut the food makes it, the more microorganisms the food will encounter. And the more microorganisms the food encounters, the more fiber that gets broken down, meaning more of the plant cells' compounds are released and reach the L-cells.

So not only is fiber food for your best health ally (gut bacteria), but it is also the packaging that brings the plant's compounds to where they can help the body produce GLP-1.

Because the wall of whole plant cells can only be broken down by your gut microbes, the cell's nutrients are not released until they reach the areas of the intestine where the microorganisms are most densely concentrated. Because things also take time in the microbial world, it takes a large number of microorganisms—solid teamwork between microbes that can do different things—before the nutrients from the plant cells are unpacked.

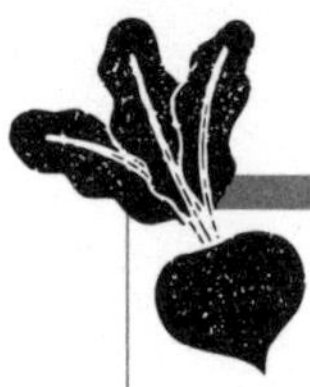

THE STRUCTURE OF FOOD IS IMPORTANT

On the left side of illustration 5, you see the refined nutrients that are "digested" or (in the case of ultra-processed foods) isolated from the natural plant structure by the food industry. When you consume these foods, the nutrients are already absorbed by the time they reach the upper part of the gut—simply because they are not wrapped in the fiber envelope the plant cell is packaged in.

Pictured on the right are the nutrients in the plant's fiber envelope, and here a good deal of teamwork is required by the gut's microorganisms to enable digestion and health-promoting biology. Think of the plant cell as a repository (or slow-release tablet) of nutrients that can make it all the way down to the areas of the gut where the GLP-1-producing gut cells are most densely concentrated. The nutrients from the plant cells make it farther down the gut only if they are inside the envelope and if the envelope is slowly broken down by the gut microbes.

So all indications suggest that the body is designed to eat food that needs to be thoroughly digested to ensure that the body's innate health mechanisms have space to work.

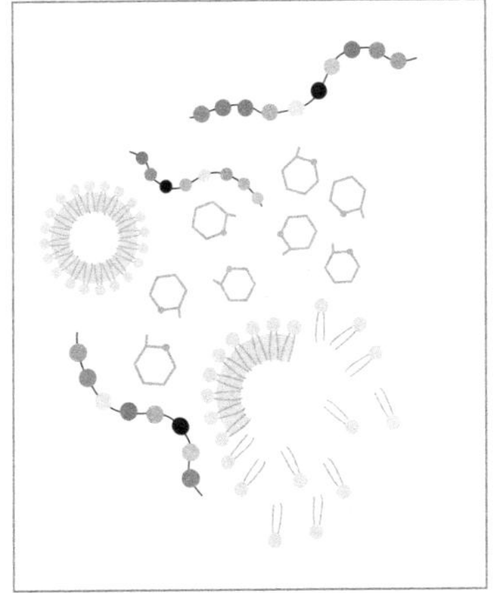

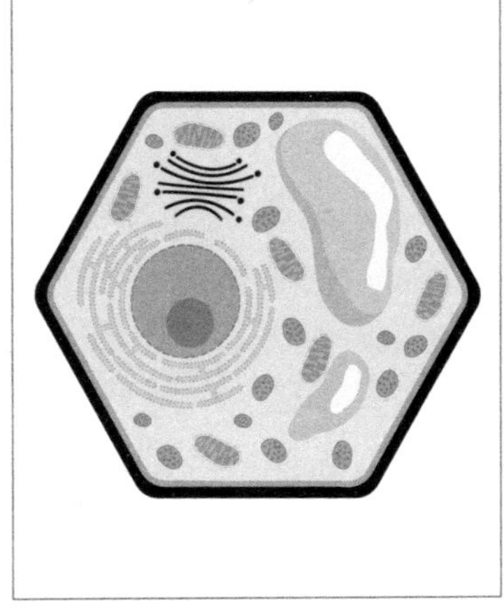

REFINED NUTRIENTS

Fully processed food—for example, refined starch and sugar (unpacked from the plant cell by the food industry)—is absorbed in the upper part of the gut and doesn't reach the intestinal flora and the L-cells farther down the digestive system.

UNPROCESSED WHOLE PLANT CELLS

Phytochemicals and nutrients in the plant cell have to be unpacked from the fiber wall and the cell structure in tandem with gut bacteria.

This process doesn't start until food makes it farther down the small intestine. So when we eat unprocessed, fiber-packed, plant-based food, think of it as creating a shortcut between the stomach and the GLP-1-laden small intestine.

Therefore it is critical for us to have a diet with lots of different nutrients, vitamins, minerals, and phytochemicals. Perhaps even more important is that all these taste-receptor activators (I know, it doesn't exactly roll off the tongue) make it to where they need to do their work. In other words, you should consider the plant cell a treasure chest filled with gold, to which only the gut microbes hold the key. Once they have unlocked the chest, the gold—in the form of nutrients, carbohydrates, fat, protein, and phytochemicals—spills out and touches the surface of the L-cells, which are ready to send GLP-1 into the bloodstream. This is also the main argument for why ultra-processed foods—even those that have a decent nutritional content low in calories—do not trigger the same health mechanisms in the body as whole, unprocessed plant cells. In processed foods, the lid is left wide open, which is why all the gold, likely of a rather poor quality, spills out the moment the chest enters the gut. Since the microorganisms do not have the key at hand, the L-cells are left to slumber in peace, and your natural GLP-1 is not released into your body.

What does this mean for the way we think about nutrition?

If natural weight loss is the goal, or if we're looking to supplement the benefits of weight-loss drugs, we need to move away from focusing on food's nutritional content and instead focus on food's nutritional *packaging,* which ensures that we both feed the gut microbes and benefit from the body's own weight-loss hormones. All this while simultaneously getting the nourishment we need for creating slow-burning energy, supplying the building blocks for your cells, and supporting the signaling molecules into the body.

You've probably already worked out that gut microbes do not work for free. While they are unpacking flavor compounds and nutrients from the plant cell, they snatch up some of your calories for themselves. This means that a low-calorie diet can be good for you and your body when your food consists of vegetables, while a low-calorie diet can go completely wrong when it only consists of fully processed "light" products that never even see the shadow of a gut microbe—or gut bacterium (we have many names for the things we love).

If you're feeling confused, don't worry, more explanations are coming. I assure you that the information in this book will offer you a new way of thinking, one that will make your life much easier.

ULTRA-PROCESSED FOOD

First, let's define unprocessed food, or food you can find at the supermarket in its original state. Food in this category is usually produce, and the many plant cells in produce all contain a cell wall made of fiber.

This cell wall is destroyed when food is ultra-processed by the food industry. It may not be surprising that I'm no fan of ultra-processed food, but it's still important to discuss. First, let's break down what makes a food count as ultra-processed.

In ultra-processed food, the fiber envelope is thrown in the trash, so the nutrients never reach the L-cells in the lower part of your gut, and at the same time—as you read in the previous description—ultra-processed food is often packed with starch in order to reestablish a structure, while additives, sugar, salt, and flour are also added. Is that good for you and your body? In the vast majority of cases, the answer is a loud and resounding NO! And now, let's take a look at the world of laboratory animals, where the effects of ultra-processed food are quickly seen.

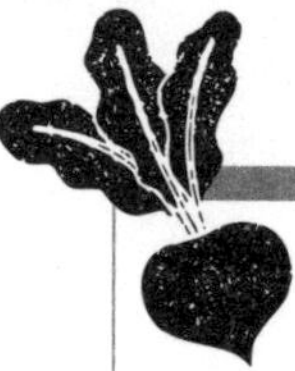

ULTRA-PROCESSED FOOD

Ultra-processed food has little in common with the food we have historically eaten.

While your ancestors probably ate unprocessed food that came—possibly with a single intermediary—directly from the farmer, the gardener, or the fisher, ultra-processed food is created by industrial methods completely unknown to previous generations.

These processes could include extrusion, where the manufacturer changes the structure, texture, taste, and color of the foods. This could include shaping, chemical modification, or hydrogenation, which makes liquid and unsaturated fat more solid. In addition, ultra-processed food often contains ingredients that, under normal circumstances, you would not find in your own kitchen.

Most often they contain a lot of sugar, salt, and starch, along with artificial sweeteners and additives. In addition, you will find ingredients like guar gum, maltodextrin, polydextrose, aspartame, xylitol, sodium carboxymethyl cellulose, and emulsifiers, while fiber and vitamins may also be added.

ALL CREATURES NEED FIBER

Research shows that if you give laboratory animals a low-fiber diet (an ultra-processed meal with no cell structures), things go very wrong:

- The digestive tract becomes smaller.

- There are fewer L-cells.

- Not only does the smaller intestinal area have fewer cells, but there is also far less GLP-1 in the rest of the gut.

- The intestine becomes permeable, so components from the food and the gut microbes seep into the body, where they can cause damage, including inflammation.

The gut becomes leaky likely because GLP-1 is typically released with its cousin, GLP-2. I've not described GLP-2 in depth yet; simply note that GLP-2, among other things, preserves the gut's barrier function by producing strong, new barrier cells. The effect is so drastic that the gut actually grows bigger when you inject GLP-2 into laboratory animals and patients with reduced bowel function.

The problem with ultra-processed, predigested food, then, is not simply that we do not trigger enough satiety hormones, but we also lose important maintenance of the intestines, which has proven to be far more crucial than we ever realized—until recently.

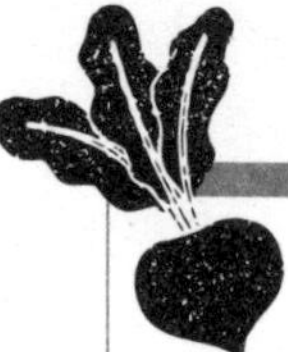

THE NOVA CLASSIFICATION

In 2009, a new framework, the Nova classification, appeared for the first time in scientific literature. The Nova classification divides foods into four distinct categories, which can be a brilliantly simple tool when you're deciding whether to eat certain foods.

GROUP 1:
UNPROCESSED OR MINIMALLY PROCESSED FOOD

Unprocessed food like fresh produce, meat, and eggs.

Minimally processed food is natural food that has been subjected to only minimal processes such as drying, freezing, or packaging, or the inedible parts have been removed.

GROUP 2:
PROCESSED CULINARY INGREDIENTS

Ingredients derived from Group 1 foods that are commonly used in cooking. Examples include salt, sugar, butter, cooking oil, seeds, nuts, and honey. These are typically free of additives, although some may include added vitamins or minerals.

GROUP 3:
PROCESSED FOOD

Food that has been produced by mixing foods from Groups 1 and 2, including salted nuts, cheese, canned fruit and vegetables, canned fish in oil, homemade bread, and beer.

These processes involve different methods of preparing and preserving the quality of the food, aiming to improve the shelf life and quality of Group 1 foods. Additives such as antioxidants and preservatives may appear.

GROUP 4:
ULTRA-PROCESSED FOOD

Industrial products with a lot of ingredients. A number of these ingredients would be unusual to find in your kitchen. Examples include coloring agents, emulsifiers, and thickeners. These are often produced by combining several methods or through extensive processing. Foods in this group include packaged bread, crackers, pastries, soft drinks, chocolate, ice cream, hot dogs, and burgers.

Ultra-processed food can be classified as industrially produced products. They consist of chemically altered substances from raw materials such as modified starch and protein isolates, which are combined with additives to give them the right flavor, consistency, appearance, and shelf life. Products include instant mashed potatoes, liver pâté, and muffins packaged in plastic.

CORRELATION BETWEEN ULTRA-PROCESSED FOOD AND MODERN-LIFESTYLE DISEASES

If we continue down this path and look at studies on ordinary people, I can put it rather bluntly: There is a strong correlation between the availability of ultra-processed food and the prevalence of obesity, as well as that of at least thirty different illnesses, including cancer, psychiatric diagnoses, respiratory diseases, circulatory diseases, infertility, diseases of the gastrointestinal tract, and a wide range of metabolic disorders, such as type 2 diabetes. Furthermore, there is also a strong correlation between the availability of ultra-processed food and the risk of premature death from *anything*.

Let me give you some figures. If you increase the quantity of ultra-processed food you consume by 10 percent, you increase your risk of metabolic disorders by 4 percent. Some studies show that on average, between 50 and 75 percent of our food falls into the ultra-processed category.

Read those two sentences again. And once again. In other words: Few things have a worse impact on human health than ultra-processed food. We can look at the downsides in two ways:

Is the increased risk of disease due to all the things you *get* from eating ultra-processed food—lots of calories, rapid blood sugar spikes, and outsized cravings demanding more and more? Or is the risk due to all the things you do *not* get from ultra-processed food—no helpful gut hormones, no happy well-nourished gut microbes, and no robust regulation of appetite, metabolism, or satiety?

While we don't have definitive proof that it's one over the other, my best guess is that it's a combination of both problems—and that they each exacerbate the other.

Over the following pages, aided by illustrations and text boxes, I'll explain why, whatever you do, you should do your best to avoid filling your plate with ultra-processed food. I recognize that this is not always possible, whether because of the food available in your community or what you're able to afford. Or, sometimes you just want to enjoy a burger with some friends. In those cases, I urge you to consider it an indulgence, balanced out by plenty of Group 1, unprocessed foods.

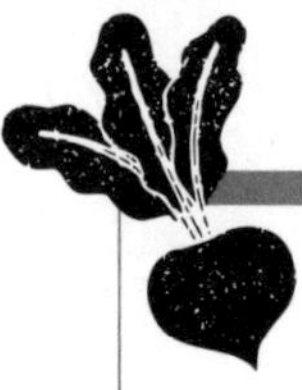

YOUR RELATIONSHIP WITH PROCESSED AND UNPROCESSED FOOD

Nutrients from the food you eat have to be delivered to where the L-cells are situated in order to be effective. Whole plant cells make it past the upper part of the digestive tract and only leak out flavor compounds and nutrients when the friendly gut bacteria break down the fiber wall of the plant cells. At this point, you're able to share the nutrients with the microbes, who thank you by sending stimulants to your immune system, your central nervous system, and your L-cells, which then deliver the GLP-1 package.

Think of the plant cell's outer layer as packaging that allows you to create a healthy journey between the stomach and small intestine, as we saw in illustration 2.

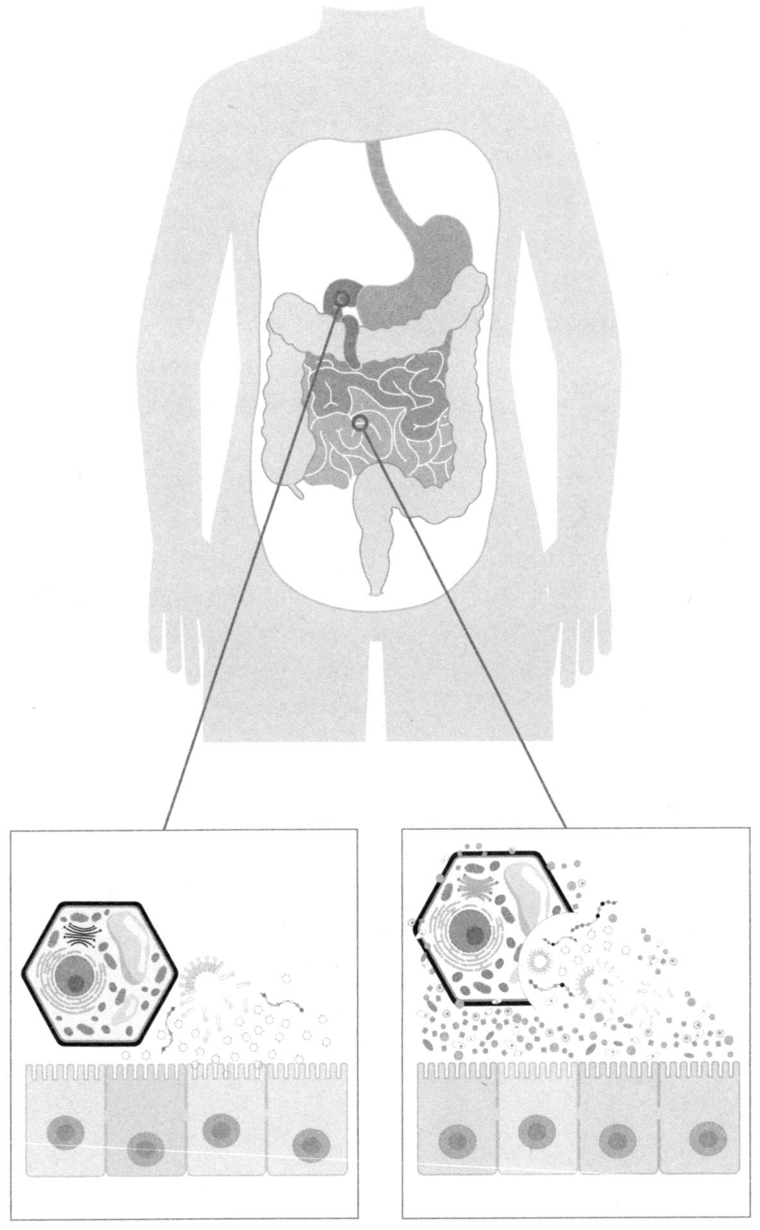

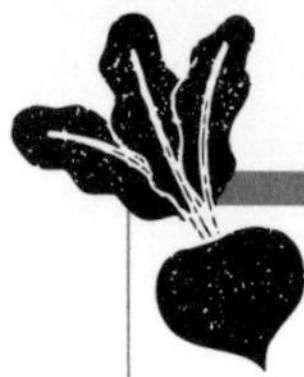

ULTRA-PROCESSED FOOD

All ultra-processed food is industrially processed to create a product that sells well. The packaging can often advertise the use of "real" food, giving you a false sense of security about what you're eating.

The following is a list of foods that are typically ultra-processed.

1. **Protein and granola bars**
    These bars often contain processed fibers and proteins as well as zero-calorie sweeteners, plus additives and preservatives.

2. **Bread**
    Certain types of bread, especially those packaged in plastic and already sliced, may contain emulsifiers, sugar, modified starch, additives, preservatives, and vegetable gums. In addition, a lot of bread is baked using flour where the grain is processed into almost pure starch.

3. **Flavored yogurt**
    Flavored yogurt often contains additives like thickeners, artificial flavorings, and preservatives to maintain shelf life.

4. **Ready-made sauces and spice mixes**
    These products often contain thickening and coloring agents, additives, preservatives, and flavor enhancers.

5. **Breakfast cereals and drinks**

   Many breakfast cereals and drinks marketed as healthy
   may contain ingredients such as coloring agents and
   maltodextrin, as well as many common additives and
   preservatives.

6. **Processed meat**

   Prepackaged cold cuts, sausages, and bacon may
   contain emulsifiers, thickening agents, additives,
   preservatives, and modified starch.

7. **Margarine and plant-based butters**

   Margarine and plant-based butters often contain
   emulsifiers, additives, preservatives, and coloring agents.

8. **Soft drinks and energy drinks**

   These beverages are typically packed with sugar,
   preservatives, and artificial additives.

9. **Plant-based "milks"**

   Many milk alternatives contain emulsifiers, vegetable
   gums, preservatives, and flavor additives.

10. **Certain meat substitutes**

   These products, which include "plant-based" steaks,
   meatballs, and patties, often (but do not always) contain
   a lot of starch, sugar, flavoring agents, and additives
   and preservatives.

Look at the list of ingredients on the label and judge whether it's
something you want to eat (and share with your gut bacteria).

The sick thing—and yes, I do mean it when I say "sick"—is that most of us have been manipulated so much by the food industry that ultra-processed food now seems natural, while natural food seems weird.

Instead of heading straight for the crunchy, salty, and fatty options in the supermarket aisles, turn your shopping habits upside down and start with the following items when you go shopping:

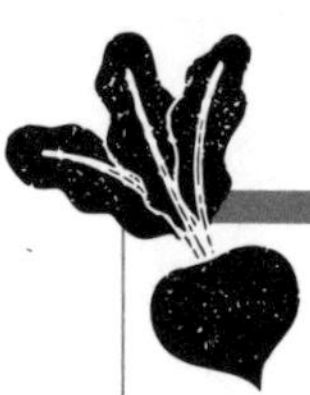

CABBAGE AND OTHER FIBROUS VEGETABLES

Broccoli, Brussels sprouts, cauliflower, lettuce, kale, cabbage, asparagus, spinach, and more.

VEGETABLES

Squash, onions, leeks, mushrooms, tomatoes, cucumbers, celeriac, peas, eggplant, celery, beets, artichokes, parsnips, herbs, chiles, and more.

FRUIT AND BERRIES

Apples, pears, bananas, blueberries, grapes, melon, strawberries, and more.

PULSES AND LENTILS

Black beans, snow peas, black-eyed peas, soybeans, lentils, and more.

NUTS AND SEEDS

Hazelnuts, cashews, walnuts, almonds, pumpkin seeds,
pine nuts, sunflower seeds, sesame seeds, chia seeds,
flaxseed, psyllium husks, and more.

FATS

Olive oil, canola oil, coconut milk,
avocado, tahini, and more.

DAIRY PRODUCTS

Cheese, skyr, yogurt, milk, cream,
kefir, and more (but watch out for additives,
sugar, artificial sweeteners, etc).

MEAT, EGGS, FISH, AND SHELLFISH

Salmon, cod, chicken, beef, lamb, game,
shrimp, mussels, eggs, and more.

PLANT PROTEINS

Tofu, tempeh, concentrated protein powder
(but watch out for additives, sugar, etc.), and more.

GRAINS AND RICE

Rice, oats, certain flourless breads made with
whole grains, seeds and kernels, and more.

The list of whole foods may seem overwhelming, not least because it is not exhaustive. Fortunately, there is a way to make incorporating healthy eating into your life easier. We can, for example, divide all foods into four categories based on carbohydrate content and the degree of processing. You can find my simple food breakdown on pages 52–53.

When we look at the effects of naturally occurring GLP-1 in the body, it's a little more difficult to see which positive effects come from the GLP-1 alone and which come from all the other positive benefits of the foods and lifestyle that lead us to produce GLP-1. Let's look at that a little more in the next chapter.

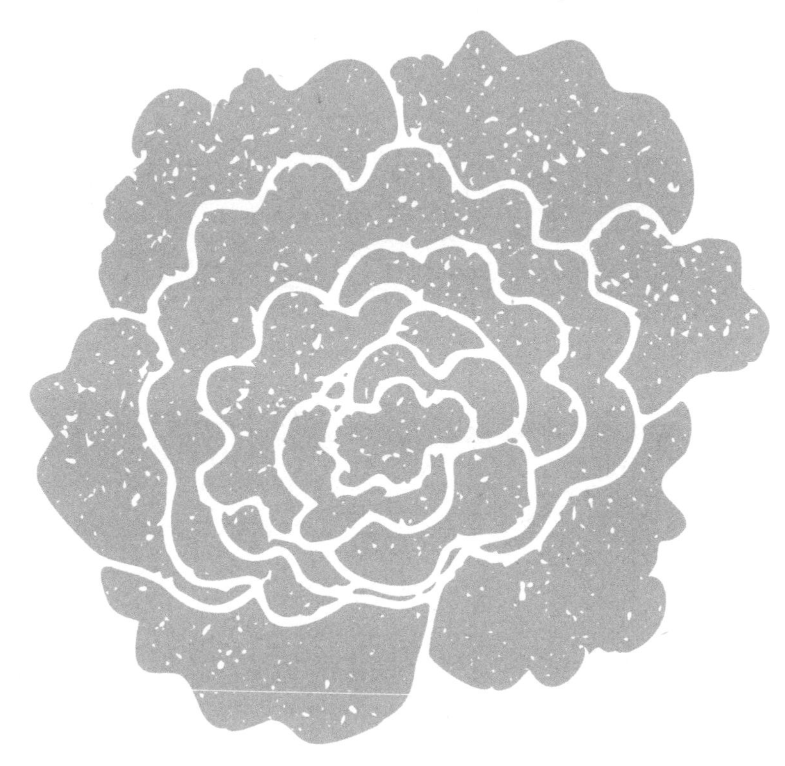

Chapter 6

The scientific dilemma

In previous chapters, we have looked at how GLP-1 forms naturally, and how the body can put extra GLP-1 to work, either when detours in the intestines are created or when you eat foods that—in tandem with the microorganisms in the intestines—distribute the many nutrients throughout the entire digestive system and to the parts of the gut where the L-cells are most densely situated. I also proposed that regular exercise and intervals between meals can promote the formation of GLP-1.

Before we move on to even deeper insight in the section about the impact of GLP-1 on the body, you should know about the scientific dilemma standing in the way of "bio-logic" being a genuine partner in a healthy world. But what the heck is biologic?

In short, I use the word *biologic* to describe a biological logic. You can think of it as the GPS showing you a safe route to a healthier life. Your entire biologic can be summed up in ten points:

1. Excess sugar in the blood is unwelcome because sugar reacts with your proteins, stresses your cells, activates

your immune response, reduces the body's ability to burn fat, messes with your appetite, and decreases the ability to remove excess sugar from the blood.

2. By working with sugar's timeline of release in the blood and the body's ability to store that sugar, you can change the risk of excess sugar in the blood. The release time is affected by both the amount and degree of refinement of carbohydrate-rich foods, while the storage capacity depends on your blood sugar history and how much you use your muscles. The risk of excess sugar in the blood is also affected by when you eat, when you exercise, and when you sleep.

3. You have to work together with the body's micro-organisms: If you feed them unprocessed vegetables, grains, and seeds, the microorganisms pay you back with nutrients, vitamins, a balanced immune response, and stabilization of your appetite and blood sugar.

4. By eating unprocessed foods, you stimulate the formation of hormones in your intestines, create satiation and satisfaction, and stabilize your blood sugar.

5. Stable blood sugar stabilizes your weight and your energy level. At the same time, higher energy levels and falling weight further stabilize your blood sugar.

6. Sugar content is often related to the level of processing that a certain food has undergone, and sugar

consumption spurs sugar cravings. This is a process you can control.

7. If you feel tired and lack energy and are craving something sweet or salty, what I like to call "exercise snacks"—brief moments of physical activity—can often replace chocolate and other processed snacks.

8. Elevated blood sugar is self-perpetuating, but it is possible to break the negative spiral.

9. Stable blood sugar is positively self-perpetuating—and a positive spiral can be set in motion much faster than actual weight loss.

10. Stabilization of the blood sugar has great and often overlooked health potential, which can replace downward disease spirals with upward health spirals.

With all that established, the scientific question is whether healthy unprocessed foods, exercise, and intervals between meals produce weight loss, or GLP-1 triggers these actions.

The answer is that it is a combination of both, and figuring out the extent to which the effect comes from one or the other is not a trivial matter. We can turn to science for answers, but note that you never get the same scientific certainty in lifestyle studies where people change their diet and activity levels as you do with clinical drug studies.

In the pharmaceutical industry, when we talk about the extent to which the patient actually takes their medication in the way it is described on the label, we refer to it as *compliance*. Although life often gets in the way and we do not always take medicine correctly, it is easier for the test subject to inject a pen in the abdomen once a week than to alter their diet drastically from the 50 to 75 percent consumption of ultra-processed food that has become the new normal in many countries.

Also, those who take part in trials meant to test the effects of dietary changes alone, where you are served whole foods three times a day for free and at the same time receive lots of attention and personalized health targets over the course of a trial, often choose to return to their previous lifestyle when the trial period has ended—meaning that the takeaways from those trials cannot always be extrapolated to average daily life.

In other words: Your desire for weight loss + your willpower + your extra efforts in the kitchen + your understanding of which foods are best for you and why + all the temptations that surround your daily life can't be compared to your desire for weight loss + your compliance when all you have to do is give yourself a small injection once a week.

This was quite a digression on how difficult it is to conduct food trials on people, but the dilemma is even greater. Semaglutide and other GLP-1 replicas have a much longer shelf life than the body's natural GLP-1, meaning that a dose of semaglutide can reach the entire body. Natural GLP-1, on the other hand, breaks down quickly as it travels from the L-cells and around the body.

In order to understand the natural weight-loss hormone better, researchers have attempted to inject an equal quantity of GLP-1 and other gut hormones into people who are obese as was measured in patients who had undergone the bariatric surgery from illustration 2.

Researchers observed that the trial subjects injected with the hormones ate 30 percent less than their normal dietary volume. So, in addition to the fact that patients who underwent bariatric surgery had a small stomach with less room for large meals, as described earlier, the research showed that GLP-1 adds to the weight-loss effects.

Despite continuing research—as far as I know—there is no better explanation for why the weight-loss surgeries in question have such a big effect on GLP-1 level and appetite than this: The operations result in considerably more minimally digested food reaching the small intestine.

If you want to know exactly how much of your appetite regulation and weight loss is due to the GLP-1 your body produces, you'll have to be patient for a few more years. To measure whether the body's natural GLP-1 results in 10 percent, 50 percent, or 90 percent of your weight loss, a medication blocking the effects of GLP-1 has to be developed first. Once that drug exists, a study can be conducted in which two groups of people eat and live the same way, but with one group taking the GLP-1-blocking medication. Only then can the degree to which GLP-1 affects appetite regulation and weight loss be ascertained.

In the following chapters, I will share some of the knowledge we have about GLP-1, and we will look at the similarities and differences between the drugs that mimic GLP-1 and the body's own wonder hormone.

Chapter 7

The GLP-1 peptide

We have spent the first part of the book describing how GLP-1 is produced and released from L-cells in the gut. We have also learned how we can transport the nutrients that release GLP-1 into the part of the gut where GLP-1 is hidden in the L-cells. Now we'll move one step further.

We are going to take a closer look at what GLP-1 actually is and how it is distributed to different places in the body. In short, to function, it attaches itself to the GLP-1 receptors on cell surfaces and triggers a biological chain reaction. After a number of intermediate steps, this chain reaction leads to lowering your blood sugar, resulting in reduced appetite and lower weight and having a radical effect on all the conditions aggravated by high blood sugar, obesity, and ultra-processed food. But I'm getting ahead of myself. Let's start with what it is all about.

GLP-1 is a *peptide*. Peptides are basically proteins—just a little smaller—but while proteins consist of long chains of amino acids, GLP-1 consists of a short chain of just thirty-one amino acids. These amino acids are held together like beads on a string in a particular order and with a particular type of chemical bond that we call the *peptide bond* or the *amide bond.*

Peptides have an important function in the body, where some act as hormones and neurotransmitters that communicate between cells and control a range of processes. The formula for the amino acid sequence in the body's own peptides and proteins can be read in your DNA, and GLP-1 has an identical sequence of amino acids in every person. When the L-cell has read your DNA and produced lots of GLP-1 peptides, they are stored in a small pocket in the L-cell and are released from there when the cell is triggered to do so. So GLP-1 is disseminated into the space around the digestive system, where it can diffuse— that is, move—into the bloodstream. So lesson number one on protein chemistry should be a closed chapter, making hormones more discernible to you.

COLLABORATION GOES BOTH WAYS

When GLP-1 is put to work, it impacts the body. But the body also impacts GLP-1. The fate of GLP-1 can go one of three ways:

- The body breaks down GLP-1 before it has managed to have an impact on the body.

- GLP-1 attaches itself to the surface of adjacent gut cells, immune cells, circulatory cells, or nerve endings and starts a biological chain reaction there.

- GLP-1 is carried by the blood to more distant regions, where it can work on other cells and nerves than those found locally surrounding the gut.

In any event, the body's natural GLP-1 has a short life span. If it makes it into the bloodstream, only half of the peptides will have survived after one or two minutes. With one of the most rapid degradation processes, the first two amino acids of the GLP-1 chain are cut off. And although most of the GLP-1 still remains, the peptide can't work without those two. The body can also cut away the last amino acid rather quickly, but it is a far gentler impairment, so it does not have as big an impact.

When GLP-1, or the aforementioned amputated versions of GLP-1, has passed into the bloodstream, it will be further degraded until finally it is sent further into the greater circulation by your kidneys.

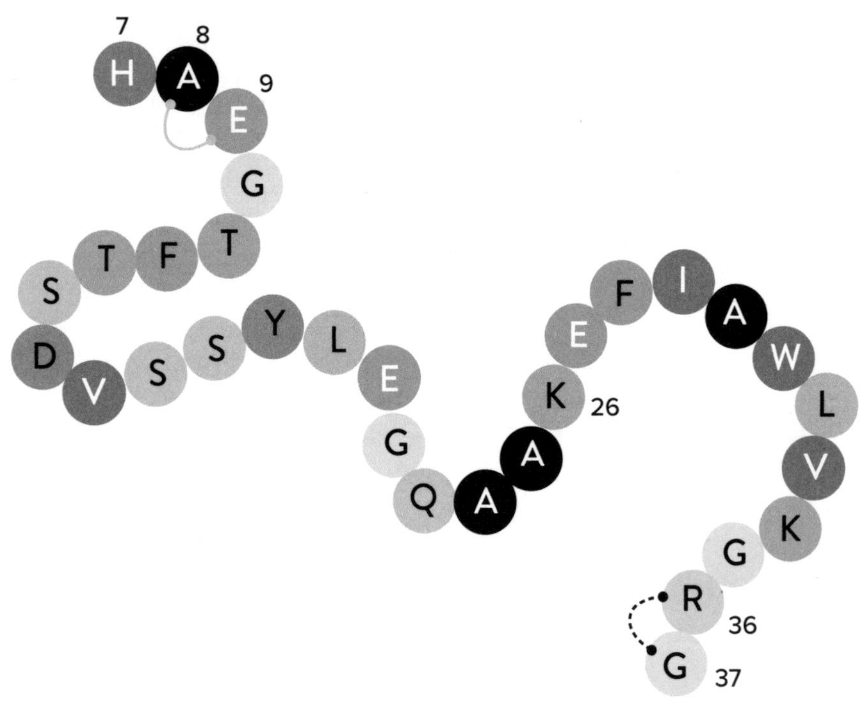
7
8
H
A
9
E
G
T
F
T
S
Y
D
V
S
S
L
E
G
Q
A
A
K
26
E
F
I
A
W
L
V
K
G
R
36
G
37

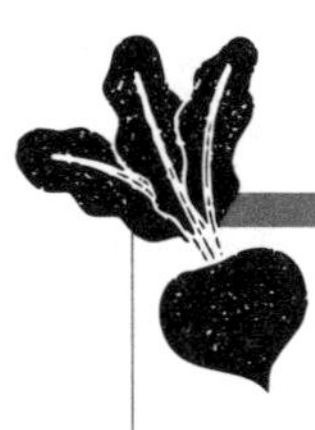

THE GLP-1 PEPTIDE—
A STRING OF AMINO ACIDS

GLP-1 is a peptide consisting of a chain of thirty-one amino acids in a particular order. The order of the amino acids is dictated by the body's DNA. You can think of the peptide molecule as a string of beads that can be twisted slightly in different directions. We designate amino acids using letters that uniquely describe which amino acid we are talking about and what it can do.

A and **E** (numbers 8 and 9) are holding hands for dear life. It is best if they do not let go, because then GLP-1 no longer works. **R** and **G** (numbers 36 and 37) hold hands loosely, but if **G** waves goodbye to the rest of the peptide, GLP-1 can still attach to the receptor and work there.

K (number 26) can carry something rather exceptional and valuable. This is where Novo Nordisk has figured out how to create the medication semaglutide.

The strings of amino acids in GLP-1 and semaglutide are 94 percent identical, but while the body's own GLP-1 disappears from the bloodstream after around two minutes, half of the semaglutide molecules live for more than 165 hours—about a week—because the talented researchers at Novo Nordisk have cleverly slowed the breakdown of the peptide!

If you wonder why the first amino acid in GLP-1 is designated as number 7 instead of number 1, you can read the entire story about how GLP-1 was first discovered in the book *The Story of GLP-1* (*Historien om GLIP-1*) by Jens Juul Holst (FADL, 2024).

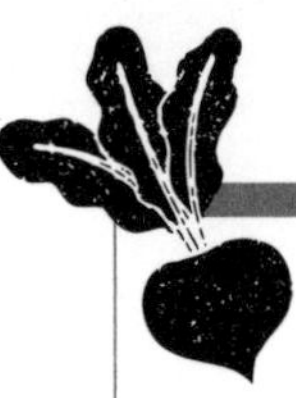

HURRAH FOR ALL THE TALENTED RESEARCHERS

Generous and mutual collaboration between talented researchers at universities and in the pharmaceutical industry has led to the groundbreaking understanding of how natural GLP-1 works in the body, its effects, and its potential as a medication.

One person in particular that my fellow Danes can be proud of is Professor Jens Juul Holst. He is a genius and a pioneer who deserves all due respect for his research into GLP-1. Other brilliant junior and senior researchers in the pharmaceutical industry and at universities around the world deserve similar respect. But Jens has done something rather exceptional: He has shared his knowledge with people whose skills differ from his own, and he has established fruitful research collaborations between university researchers and the pharmaceutical industry.

Successful implementation following the discovery of GLP-1 has required thousands of committed researchers and developers and ideas both great and small. But most of all, it has required dedicated, unselfish teamwork to reach a common goal. Jens has also played an important part in this.

The Nobel Prize pays tribute to and rewards significant discoveries, and I am almost holding my breath while hoping that Jens will be honored. Let's all laud the great team spirit and the heated discussions that are a part of every new discovery.

Several medications attempt to mimic and reinforce the effects of natural GLP-1. They can be divided into two groups: GLP-1 analogs, which are long-acting replicas of GLP-1, and DPP4 inhibitors, which merely prevent the body's breakdown of its own GLP-1. Let's take a look at the last one first.

DPP4—like GLP-1—is made up of long chains of amino acids. But unlike the peptide GLP-1, DPP4 is a large protein composed of 766 amino acids. It is fixed to various cells in the body, but DPP4 also floats along freely in the bloodstream.

The medications that can inhibit DPP4 are small molecules you can take in tablet form because they can survive the journey through the digestive tract and find a way through the gut barrier and into the bloodstream. Here, the medications switch off the enzymes that cut off the two first amino acids of the GLP-1 molecule (see illustration 7, page 74). With that, your body's own GLP-1 gets more time to work and the effects of GLP-1 are reinforced. Clever.

Unfortunately, DPP4 also breaks down other peptides, which—unlike GLP-1—become active only once a bit of their string of amino acids has been cut off. So just like with everything else in life, nothing is ever completely black or white, good or bad. However, DPP4 inhibitors are good medications for the treatment of diabetes, and they are manufactured by several pharmaceutical companies around the world.

If we look closer at GLP-1 analogs, we can see that they are long-lasting medications that mimic the effects of natural GLP-1. In all GLP-1 replicas I know of, the molecule has been slightly altered so that DPP4 cannot amputate it. Moreover, at Novo Nordisk, they have attached a small natural fat chain to the molecule, so it is transported to every part of the body along with another large protein instead of passing straight through the filter and being secreted through the kidneys.

When GLP-1 and other peptides are taken as medications, they are normally injected into the body. This is because one of the digestive system's core functions is to break down sugar chains (carbohydrates) and amino acid chains (peptides and proteins) into sugar and amino acids, respectively. You probably remember that from illustration 4 (page 34), where we explained how amino acids, for example, can be attached to taste receptors in the gut and then ask the L-cell to release a batch of GLP-1 molecules. If you take GLP-1 as a tablet, all of the enzymes in the gut immediately break GLP-1 down into individual amino acids.

With Novo Nordisk's semaglutide, the company has created a medication that is so long-lasting that you only need to inject it into the body once a week. Research has shown that high, stable levels of GLP-1 in the blood lead to the best results.

SHOWDOWN BETWEEN GLP-1 AND SEMAGLUTIDE

On several occasions, we have seen that it is possible to combine GLP-1's positive effects with those of other natural hormones regulating weight. We call these the GLP-1 combinations. One combination product that has been marketed, for example, contains stable analogs of both GLP-1 and GIP (another weight-loss hormone from sensor cells in the gut). Zepbound (tirzepatide) from Eli Lilly contains exactly this blend. There are a number of other medications on the way using different combinations.

The future will reveal what medications combining GLP-1 with, for example, replicas of amylin, glucagon, or PYY, can do for the world's population struggling with weight.

Homemade amylin is produced and sent to work along with the body's insulin, regulating the appetite in several ways. PYY and GIP are formed in the gut's L-cells and K-cells, from where they are released along with GLP-1. These hormones similarly regulate appetite and perhaps even the sugar cravings many people experience as a strong adversary in everyday life. Glucagon is a completely natural hormone, which, on its own, goes to work between meals (if we have intervals between meals) to ensure that the blood sugar never drops too low. We will return to GIP, amylin, and PYY in Chapter 12.

Chapter 8

Where does GLP-1 work— and how

I have previously established that flavor compounds and nutrients have to reach the taste receptors on the surface of the L-cells before our food triggers a release of GLP-1. It was also emphasized that the neurotransmitter CGRP has to reach the small arteries in the muscles and all the way to the surface of the gut's L-cells to signal the release of GLP-1. The same goes for GLP-1 itself.

In order for GLP-1 to unleash all of its positive effects on blood sugar and appetite regulation, among other things, it has to reach the GLP-1 receptors on the surfaces of specific cells and attach itself to them, thereby activating the effects within the cell. We will return to the topic of which cells GLP-1 works on, but the ABCs of biology require an active molecule to be in the right place at the right time to make the difference it is meant to make.

In other words, it's no use having lots of lights in the house if you can't find the switches to turn on the lights on a dark night.

It's also no use having a giant keychain like a school janitor if none of the keys fit the lock. But where is the GLP-1 receptor (the lock) situated, how does GLP-1 (the key) reach it, and what happens when the key clicks and unlocks all the splendors inside the various cells with GLP-1 receptors on their surface?

THE KEY AND THE LOCK

As described earlier, the GLP-1 receptors are situated in specific types of cells in the body. Among other places, they sit on the so-called beta cells of the pancreas as well as in select cells in the cardiovascular system, the digestive system, the muscular system, the immune system, and the central nervous system. In other words, the receptors are rather widespread in the body and so it is not that strange that GLP-1 has many important functions.

The GLP-1 receptor sits on the surface of the cell and when GLP-1 attaches itself to the surface receptor, a chain reaction begins inside the cell. We will not go into the details of the sub-processes in this book, but you can imagine it as a small Rube Goldberg machine, with lots of crashes and bangs resulting in an extremely useful end product: biological health and weight loss, if you need it.

GLP-1 uses the same key and the same lock everywhere in the body, but whether you put the key in the lock to the bathroom, the mailbox, the front door, the patio door, the key box, or the outbuilding makes a tremendous difference. And what greets you when the door opens is also very different.

The most well-described effect of GLP-1 is what happens in the insulin-producing beta cells of the pancreas. Here the GLP-1 receptor activates a *G-protein,* triggering an enzyme that turns a small signaling molecule (ADP) into another signaling molecule (cAMP). The cAMP molecule (in the beta cell) rushes straight over and activates a new enzyme (protein kinase A), ensuring that the beta cell releases insulin.

Similar to how nutrients that arrive in the gut during digestion attach themselves to receptors, ultimately ensuring that GLP-1 is released, GLP-1 molecules that arrive with the blood in the beta cells of the pancreas ensure the fine-tuning of the amount of insulin the beta cells release during a blood sugar spike.

GLP-1 therefore has an important role in quickly removing surplus sugar from the blood after a meal, and you could rightly call GLP-1 insulin's support rider in the world's toughest cycle race. Or the teammate who passes the insulin for an easy slam dunk.

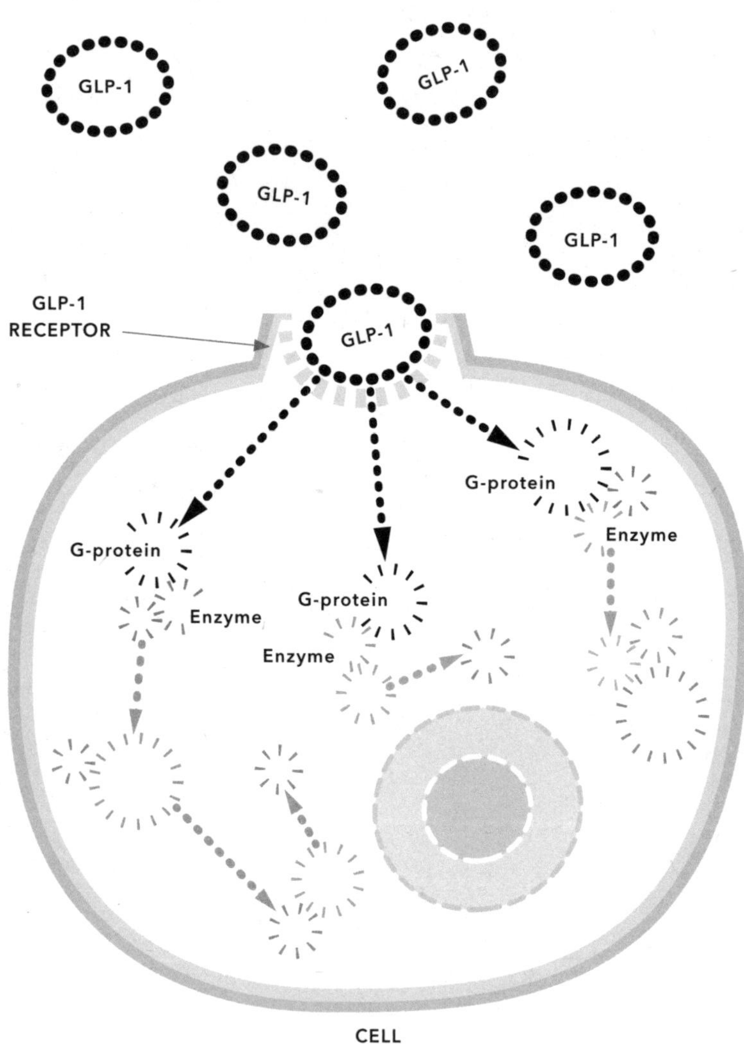

GLP-1
GLP-1
GLP-1
GLP-1
GLP-1
RECEPTOR
GLP-1
G-protein
G-protein
G-protein
Enzyme
Enzyme
Enzyme
CELL

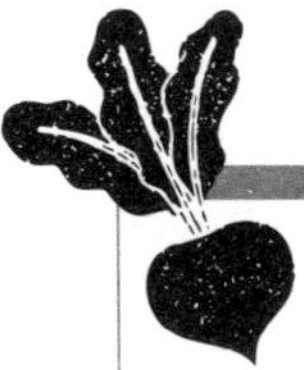

THE KEY AND THE LOCK

The GLP-1 receptor is located on the surface of particular types of cells in the body. When GLP-1 attaches itself to the GLP-1 receptor, a switch is turned on and a biological response is initiated—a small chain reaction. This response can vary in different types of cells, but as far as we know, the receptor is the same. You can compare the phenomenon with all of the light switches in your house being identical, but the lamps and lights that turn on when you flip on different switches can vary significantly in the living room, the bedroom, the bathroom, or the study.

The GLP-1 receptor—exactly like every other receptor in the body—is made up of amino acids. When GLP-1 works its way into the receptor, it rotates its string of beads a little differently, so the receptor can reach another protein inside the cell (the G protein), which then reaches an enzyme in the cell. This enzyme transforms a small signaling molecule into another small signaling molecule, and the new signaling molecule switches on a new enzyme, which in some cells ensures that insulin is released. Given this explanation, I think you'll understand why I previously compared all of this to a Rube Goldberg machine.

THE FINE-TUNING
OF TWO IMPORTANT HORMONES

In addition to GLP-1 fine-tuning the insulin levels in the pancreas's beta cells, it also influences the pancreas's alpha cells. The alpha cells are located right next to the beta cells, and their primary objective is to send the hormone glucagon to work.

In many ways, glucagon does the opposite of insulin. Whereas insulin lowers the blood sugar after a meal, glucagon ensures that the blood sugar rises a tiny bit if it gets a little too low. This is why it makes perfect sense that GLP-1 fine-tunes both insulin and glucagon in each direction. The GLP-1 receptor is the same in alpha cells and beta cells, but the chain reactions inside these cells are slightly different.

For years, researchers have discussed whether GLP-1 reaches the pancreas via the bloodstream or whether there is a small *shuttle* that helps transport active GLP-1 there. Despite this discussion—or perhaps because of it—GLP-1's effect on blood sugar is more important than it may seem here. Stable blood sugar is an important health accelerator, because a high sugar level in the blood leads to a number of problems, and because stable blood sugar decreases your appetite for sugar.

WALTZ WITH THE STOMACH

GLP-1 has important effects on the appetite, and there are at least two reasons for that.

First, GLP-1 attaches itself to receptors on the surface of muscle cells in the stomach and parietal cells. The latter are cells in the mucus membrane of the stomach that, among other things, ensure the secretion of hydrochloric acid into the stomach. When the key enters the lock here, the stomach's digestive processes and rhythmic movements are reduced, making the food stay in the stomach a little longer. When your stomach is full of food, you feel fuller.

But it doesn't stop here, because GLP-1 has other direct effects on how full you feel. This is due to its effects on the brain's own appetite-regulation center, the hypothalamus. The hypothalamus is the destination point of many different hunger and satiation signals from the nervous system, hormones, blood sugar, and so on. And in a clever way that we do not yet fully understand, the hypothalamus figures out whether the sum of all the different stimuli results in hunger or satiation. Complicated, but it is absolutely certain that GLP-1—if it makes it all the way up to the hypothalamus before it is broken down—directly influences the nerve cells in the hypothalamus.

Beyond the well-described effects on blood sugar and appetite, there is much to indicate that GLP-1 reduces the unwanted inflammation you often carry in your system when you are overweight, have long periods with too much sugar in the blood, or are missing all the good anti-inflammatory stimulants that vegetables and healthy gut microbes offer us.

Several smaller studies show the anti-inflammatory effects of GLP-1 on cells of blood vessels (known as endothelium cells), cardiac muscle cells (cardiomyocytes), immune cells (including macrophages), and fat cells. In these types of cells, there are numerous indications that the receptor activation of GLP-1 can produce signaling molecules that act a little like antioxidants, which can control an overactive immune system.

On the one hand, we have the effect on the individual cells cultivated outside the body. On the other, we have the manifestation of all these effects in the entire living body. We can therefore conclude that there is a synergy between all of the effects mentioned, which is why I call the effects a *positive health spiral.*

THE TRULY POSITIVE HEALTH SPIRAL IS CALLED INSULIN SENSITIVITY

When GLP-1 adjusts blood sugar regulation by fine-tuning insulin and glucagon, a wealth of health-promoting effects is set in motion. Stable blood sugar alone has a positive effect on appetite regulation, sugar cravings, and inflammation and, in turn, on your body's defense against obesity, cardiovascular disease, infertility, pain, dementia, and all of the other conditions we looked at earlier. So let's pause for a moment to take a closer look at blood sugar.

The way your diet affects blood sugar varies from person to person. Although the processes controlling the unpacking and breakdown of carbohydrates, the conversion of carbohydrates into sugar, and the transference of sugar from the digestive system into the bloodstream is individual and dependent on your gut flora, it is our ability to remove excess sugar from the blood that determines how much our blood sugar rises after a given meal. It is also our ability to remove excess sugar from the blood that determines how long it takes before the blood sugar returns to the level we call *fasting blood sugar.*

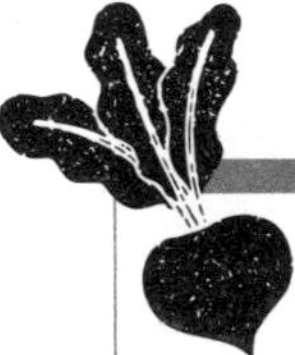

WHAT IS BLOOD SUGAR?

Blood sugar is another term for the concentration of glucose in your blood.

When you consume carbohydrates, they're broken down into sugar in the digestive system, which are absorbed by the gut, after which your blood sugar level rises. You are aware from earlier in the book that glucose also attaches to the sensors of the L-cells.

After this, the blood sugar is regulated by insulin, which directs the glucose from the blood into the muscle cells and liver cells, where it is either immediately used as energy or stored for later use. Insulin works by attaching itself to insulin receptors on the surface of particular muscle and liver cells. When the insulin receptor is activated here, it ensures that small pathways are opened, which draw excess sugar from the blood into the muscle or liver cell. In this way, your blood sugar level is lowered.

If the sugar level in your blood is too high, your healthy body releases insulin to lower it. If the blood sugar is too low, the well-functioning body releases the hormone glucagon to increase it, because the body would prefer to maintain a nice and stable blood sugar.

Fasting blood sugar is measured in mmol/L, which is a measurement of the number of sugar molecules in a liter of blood. While the normal range for fasting blood sugar varies between around 4 and 6.5 mmol/L, we have on average a fasting blood sugar of around 5.5 mmol/L, which corresponds to around 5 grams of sugar per liter, or around two sugar cubes per liter. The normal fasting blood sugar is also given in mg/dL, and a normal fasting blood glucose is less than 100 mg/dL.

Fasting blood sugar—as the name implies—is a measurement of your blood sugar when your latest meal is fully digested and the body has placed the nutrients into storage to the best of its ability.

How effectively we remove excess sugar from the blood depends on many factors, including genetics; age; the amount of muscle, brown fat, and white fat in the body; whether we have inflammation, stress, and disease in the body; how and how much we move; and what and how often we eat.

In general, the younger we are, the more muscle mass we have, the less fat around the waist, the more physical activity we do, the less inflammation we have, and the more unprocessed vegetable-rich food we eat, the more efficient the body is at removing excess sugar from the blood.

Likewise, seven to nine hours of sleep per night also has a positive effect on insulin sensitivity, because sleep ensures periods of not eating and improves your chance of having energy to move during the course of the day.

WHEN GLUCAGON IS SUPPRESSED

Let's look at the example in illustration 9 (pages 92–93). On paper, three perfectly normal carbohydrate-containing meals from the traditional carbohydrate-rich Western diet will affect the insulin level of a young, active person rather differently from that of an older, less active person.

Since a high insulin level suppresses glucagon, among other things, there will be a significant difference from person to person in when the glucagon is allowed to poke out its nose and say: "Make sugar from fat." In principle, there should be a big difference when the glucagon increases your metabolism!

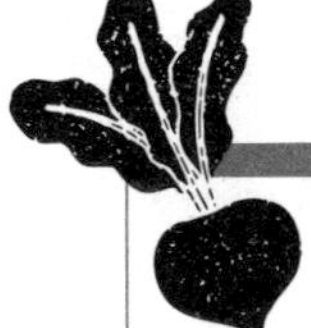

WHAT IS INSULIN SENSITIVITY?

Our ability to remove excess sugar from the blood is called *insulin sensitivity*. The faster we remove excess sugar from the blood, the higher our insulin sensitivity and carbohydrate tolerance and the lower our insulin resistance. The slower we remove sugar from the blood, the more insulin resistance, the lower insulin sensitivity, and the lower carbohydrate tolerance we have.

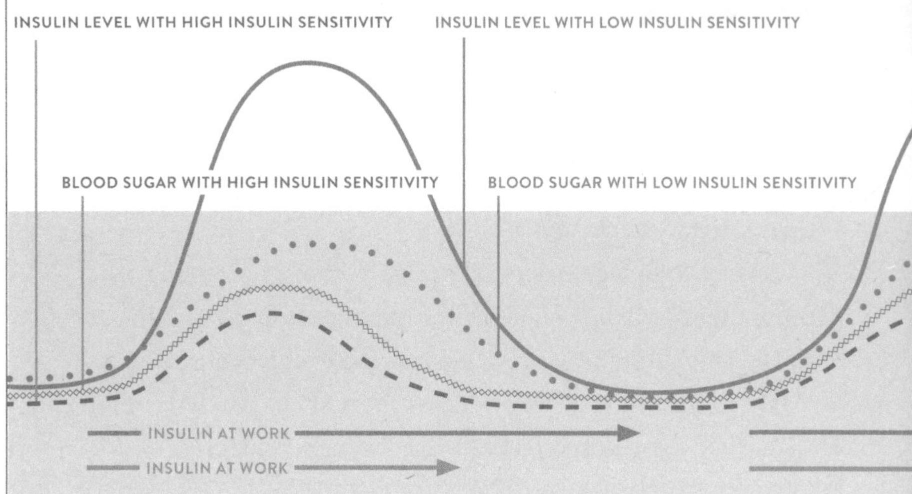

BLOOD SUGAR—NOT THE SAME FOR EVERYONE

The four curves show blood sugar and insulin levels for two people with different insulin sensitivity and sugar tolerance. It could be a younger and an older person, an inactive and an active person, one with the flu and one without—or one with a high muscle mass and one with a high fat mass.

The two people consume the exact same meals, but as the curves show, the amount of sugar and insulin in the blood differs.

In the solid and dotted lines (the insulin-resistant person), the blood sugar and insulin levels are higher, and it takes more time before the sugar and insulin levels return to the starting point after each of the three meals. In addition, insulin also works longer in the body with the insulin-resistant person than the person who is insulin-sensitive (note the arrows below the curves).

In the case of the person who is sugar-tolerant and insulin-sensitive, during meals (the dashed and diamond curves), excess sugar in the blood is quickly drawn away from the blood, after which glucagon can allow glucose molecules from the liver back into the blood as required.

Since the blood sugar increase is higher in the insulin-resistant person, and because insulin's work takes place for a longer period after the meal, there will be less time from when insulin disappears to when the next meal is consumed, when insulin has to go back to work. In principle, this means that the insulin-resistant body does not listen very well the next time insulin shouts its "Get sugar away from the blood" command.

Here the alarm bells are ringing loud and clear! However, the insulin-resistant person can achieve a blood sugar curve closer to the diamond curve of the insulin-sensitive person if they choose to eat a meal that does not contain as many (refined) carbohydrates as the typical Western diet calls for. In other words, the insulin-resistant person can regulate blood sugar through diet and muscle activity.

Whether it is then necessary to make an active effort to achieve stable blood sugar naturally depends on the health condition of the person, meaning it is fundamentally important that you understand your blood sugar. You do not necessarily have to measure it, however. Blood sugar readings are routine only for people with diabetes.

Take another quick look at the illustration. What do you think happens if the person who is insulin-sensitive and the sedentary person who is insulin-resistant each eat a piece of whole-grain bread and a couple pieces of fruit between meals three times a day?

In the insulin-resistant person, the solid line curve will remain just above the fasting blood sugar level most of the day, while the insulin-sensitive person's curve will be almost unchanged, as the small surplus of sugar in the blood is stabilized in a flash. Using a track-and-field analogy, the insulin-sensitive person's insulin is standing on the starting line, fully rested after the previous meal, waiting for its turn. For those who are insulin-resistant, however, glucagon is pacing in the starting area while insulin is still doing its lap, and when insulin, with the consumption of the bread and fruit, has to run another lap before it gets a chance to rest, the body is less responsive to insulin's instructions to remove sugar from the blood. Since insulin did not get a chance to rest, glucagon never made it out of the starting area.

Here we can conclude that the better your insulin sensitivity, the easier it is to maintain both good insulin sensitivity and a healthy weight, and the easier it is to maintain a healthy weight, the easier it is to stay insulin-sensitive and energetic, making it even easier to maintain that insulin sensitivity. This is the positive health spiral everyone would like to be in. Fortunately, it is one that you, I, and most people can return to if we have dropped out of it.

You can regain insulin sensitivity by maintaining a high level of physical activity, preserving muscle mass, ensuring that blood sugar remains normal between meals, and making sure gut hormones and microbiota have a good working relationship with lots of well-packaged plant cells.

Stable blood sugar creates good appetite regulation, which creates a healthier weight, and a healthier weight creates higher insulin sensitivity and more stable blood sugar. And there you have it. That is the ultimate positive health spiral, on top of all the work GLP-1 does on its own.

Before we proceed, we'll take another look at why it is so important to maintain stable blood sugar, so that glucagon and insulin are allowed to interact—thanks to their support rider, GLP-1.

THE BODY'S TRIPARTITE AGREEMENT

Blood sugar, insulin resistance, and inflammation directly affect one another. When the three of them are operating at stable levels, you have a really good chance of feeling well, full of energy, and healthy. When one is out of balance, it drags the others down with it.

Biologically, this makes sense. Every single moment, your body is monitoring whether it is being invaded by pathogenic bacteria or viruses. The body typically discovers the invasion by way of the receptor molecules of the immune system—think of it as the body's radar—which register unknown protein structures in the body. Imagine that the protein structures are the uniforms of the microorganisms, and that the uniforms are protein molecules dressed in sugar. We call them glycoproteins.

When the immune system's receptor molecules register foreign glycoproteins (sugar-bound proteins) in the body, the immune system is activated (that is, when there's a lot of extra sugar in the blood, the immune system is triggered). In addition to activating its disease-fighting immune cells, the immune system also sends chemical messages to your energy stores (muscle and liver cells in particular), telling them to refrain from capturing more sugar for storage; this results in even more free-roaming sugars in the bloodstream. In fact, the immune system's battle for your survival hinges on there being enough sugar for the immune system's cells to be able to combat the external invasion, which is why the cells have to ignore the messages from the insulin in the blood. This is why excess sugar can be so problematic: Not only does it trigger the immune system, but it also leads the immune system to send messages that decrease insulin sensitivity.

At this point, we have a situation with high levels of both insulin and blood sugar, along with heightened activity in the immune system—and we have muscle and liver cells that unfortunately allow the excess sugar to remain in the blood (it's not their fault; they're just doing as they're told). While the immune system battles the invader, there's no denying that it's working impressively hard. However, this configuration can be unfortunate in instances where the body's own proteins in a sugar-packed bloodstream are involuntarily coated in sugar molecules, making them resemble an invading virus or bacteria cell. If this happens, your immune system gears up to fight your own body, and you may have set the stage for exacerbating an inflammatory or autoimmune disease: arthritis, psoriasis, Crohn's disease, ulcerative colitis, Hashimoto's disease, atherosclerosis, and others.

Perhaps unsurprisingly, the best route to break out of insulin resistance is to seek out stable blood sugar by practicing all the good methods of achieving this goal. At the end of the book, I will offer my best tricks, including explanations on how to best ensure stable blood sugar, while simultaneously exploiting all the positive health effects, direct and indirect, of the gut microbes and GLP-1.

Chapter 9

Your body's own fuel-efficient engine

Let's conduct a little thought experiment. Imagine that your body has an engine that automatically burns off all excess energy. In addition, imagine that all the excess energy you consume does not go directly to your waist. Imagine that all the energy simply runs out of your body via a state-of-the-art exhaust pipe.

Doesn't that sound like a beautiful dream? It may in fact be more than a dream, because a lot of research indicates that your body has such a pipe. "Then why isn't it working?" you might grumble impatiently to yourself.

If we do in fact have such an exhaust pipe, its smooth functioning is blocked by modern lifestyles. Now I'm not saying I want us to return to the Stone Age, but in our modern world, generally speaking, the engine doesn't have any way to expel the exhaust, and since the hormones that should help direct that exhaust toward the exhaust pipe are simultaneously held back by ultra-processed food, the exhaust pipe is equally out of commission. The challenge lies in the fact that science is still not entirely certain of how best to connect the engine to the pipe, or to unblock the pipe, so to speak.

BROWN FAT

If you've never heard of brown fat before, you're excused because it is only in recent years that knowledge of this particular type of fat has really come into the public eye.

The abbreviation for brown fat is BAT, which stands for *brown adipose tissue*. Brown fatty tissue is distinctly different from white fatty tissue (WAT, *white adipose tissue*), which primarily stockpiles energy in the form of fat droplets.

BAT is brown in color because there are a lot more small blood vessels in brown fatty tissue, and because these fat cells have many more iron-rich mitochondria than white fat. Enough about the color—you can't see it anyway. White fatty tissue is far more common.

Unlike white fat, brown fat specializes in converting energy into heat through *non-shivering thermogenesis*. This thermal process is particularly important for sustaining body temperature in newborns, but in cold regions of the globe, people of all ages benefit from it.

Whereas white fat often gathers around your buttocks, thighs, and stomach, brown fat is primarily found in areas around the neck, along the spine, around the kidneys, and by the heart. Although the amount of BAT in our bodies is small, its ability to burn calories is significant in relation to its size.

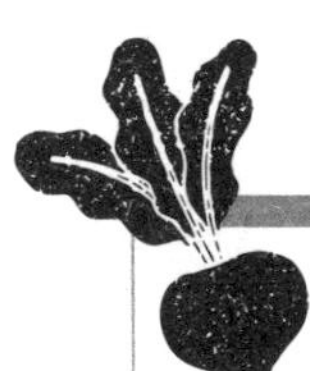

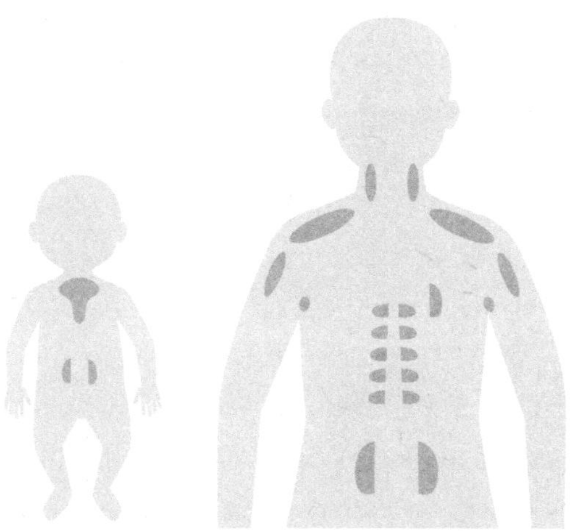

BROWN FAT

Here you can see where newborns and adults have their small reserves of healthy brown fat. We develop brown fat in the embryonic stage, and brown fat is a kind of thermostat, helping us to maintain our body temperature. At the same time, it functions as a valve that burns off energy if there is too much.

Even in the colder parts of the Northern Hemisphere, we mostly live warm, comfortable, and good lives, with waterproof clothing and central heating in our homes, and perhaps the absence of cold is one of the reasons many of us do not have much brown fat. Several different friendly hormones support us in the formation of brown fat—as do some plant chemicals. As to whether GLP-1 directly influences the formation of brown fat in particular situations, there is no agreement among scientists around the world.

Brown fat is formed in the embryonic stage, where it is developed from the same stem cells as your muscle cells. In humans, BAT is most prominent in newborns (10 to 100 grams in total), where it functions as an important source of producing heat. With age, the amount of brown fat falls to somewhere between 10 and 50 grams and becomes less active.

However, recent research has shown that adults still have some BAT, and that it can be activated and even increased in certain conditions, which indicates that white fat, in principle, can be transformed into brown fat.

TURN ON THE SWITCH

There are several ways you can either increase the amount of brown fat or simply activate it:

- **Exposure to cold:** Living in cold regions of the world is one of the most effective ways of activating brown fat. When the body is exposed to low temperatures, a particular part of your nervous system is activated that encourages BAT to produce heat. Over time, regular cold showers and going for walks in light clothing can also increase the amount of brown fat. It makes me wonder whether our well-insulated homes, warm clothing, and high-quality materials, ensuring that we never get cold, play a significant role in the current obesity epidemic that we do not fully understand but which is a result of several things. Obesity epidemic or not, however, I would be reluctant to dispense with that comfort, and I understand that others would too!

- **Physical activity:** Exercise not only increases the number of calories you burn but is proven to increase the amount of brown fat or convert white fat cells into BAT. Science is also searching for hormones released during exercise that may stimulate the production of brown fat.

- **Diet:** Certain kinds of food can affect brown fat. For example, some studies have suggested that plant chemicals from foods like chiles (capsaicin) and green tea (catechins) can activate brown fat and increase energy consumption. In addition—and now I hope you feel we've come full circle—a number of our gut hormones (for example, GIP) that are released when food makes it all the way down to the L-cells can both affect the conversion of white fat into brown fat and trigger brown fat into burning extra calories.

GLP-1 has also been proven to promote the absorption of glucose in brown fat, which increases the tissue's capacity to utilize glucose as fuel for thermogenesis—the process by which you produce heat. This contributes not only to reducing blood sugar levels but also to improving your body's overall energy balance.

Even though the amount of brown fat in adults is comparatively less than in newborns, it still plays an important role in the conversion of energy and can therefore contribute to weight control and protection against metabolic disorders such as type 2 diabetes. The growing interest surrounding brown fat in adulthood is therefore due to its potential to increase energy consumption and improve weight balance and metabolic health.

A MUSCLE IS NOT SIMPLY A MUSCLE–
A LITTLE TRICK

In the section dealing with the vital importance of insulin resistance (page 14), you read that your muscles and liver can store sugar, and that the more you use your muscles, the more inclined they are to draw excess sugar from the blood. As a result, the muscles become insulin-sensitive.

Many people (including authors of books on weight-loss hormones) sit perfectly still for nine to eleven hours every single day. When you sit still, your muscles use only about 15 percent of the energy being used by your entire body. But if you sit on a chair and raise your heels rhythmically, you activate a small 200-gram soleus muscle, which is located deep under your large calf muscle. If you sit on your bottom all day but remember to do heel raises, you reduce your blood sugar spikes after a meal by half, and likewise, the need for insulin falls by more than 50 percent.

So, simply by raising your heels, the body becomes much better at responding to insulin and much better at following its instructions. You use the same muscle when you walk or run, but what I would like to direct your attention to is that while hard muscle exercise does a lot of good, gentle muscle exercise can help you regulate blood sugar and insulin sensitivity.

It is absolutely incredible how little movement it takes to break the negative effects of inactivity.

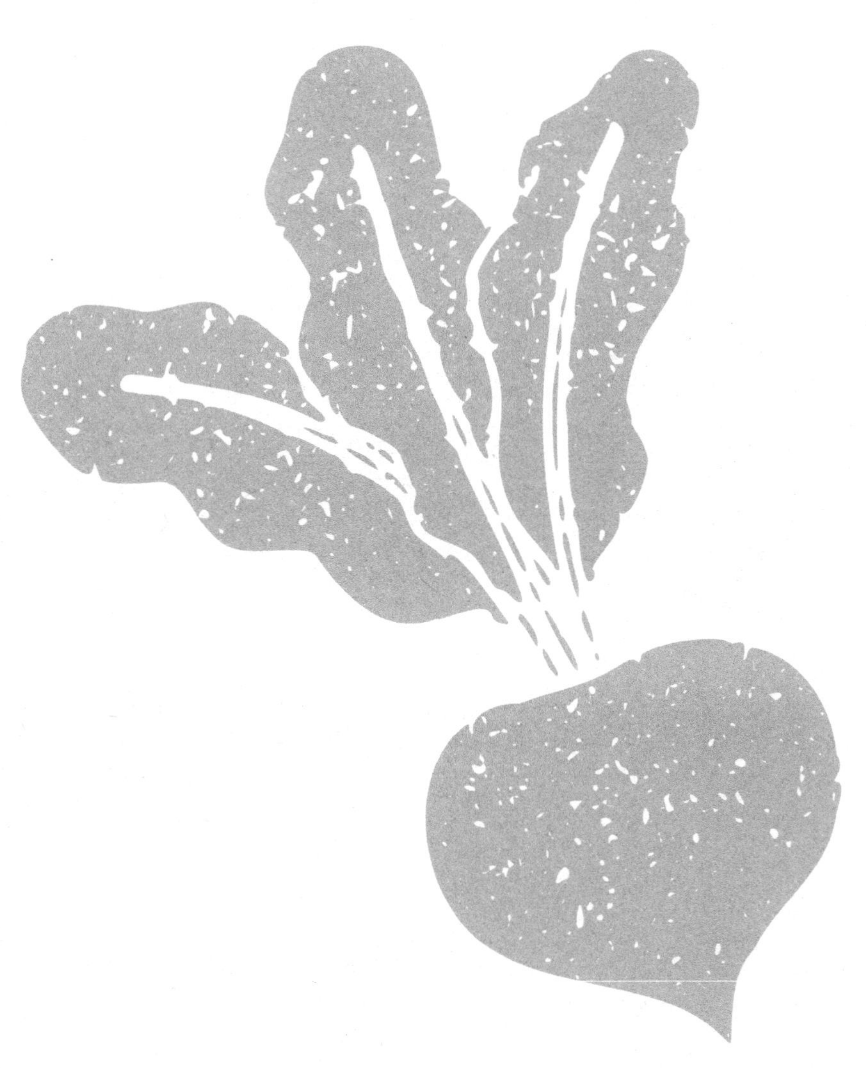

Chapter 10

GLP-1 and semaglutide— similarities and differences

The many health-promoting effects of GLP-1 are about being in the right place at the right time. I will illustrate this by looking at the similarities and differences between GLP-1 and Novo Nordisk's golden goose, semaglutide.[*]

I've included this comparison in the book because many argue that semaglutide can do things GLP-1 can't, making the body's natural weight-loss hormone inferior to the medication. Although this section may be a little technical, I hope you will benefit from reading it.

---

[*] There is a robust conversation to be had here about Eli Lilly's GLP-1 analog tirzepatide medications as well, but since my expertise is with semaglutides, I'm going to focus my attention there.

As you saw earlier (illustration 4), four things can happen with newly freed GLP-1 molecules:

- They can degrade

- They can impact local cells before they degrade

- They can impact local nerves before they degrade

- They can be transported into the bloodstream and impact areas far from the gut before they degrade

GLP-1 and semaglutide bind themselves to and activate exactly the same GLP-1 receptor. This means that both keys fit the lock, but GLP-1 is a little better at activating the receptor than semaglutide. On the other hand, semaglutide lasts longer.

As mentioned earlier, it's a matter of a certain effect requiring us to have a certain activator with the right quantity and in the right place. While semaglutide comes from a small needle injected into the fatty tissue under your skin once a week, your body's natural GLP-1 comes from the L-cells in the digestive system. Since your homemade GLP-1 lasts in the body for only a few minutes, we would expect it to work especially well locally, while semaglutide, which lasts for a week, can make it to every part of the body and go to work there.

The favorable effects we see with semaglutide come on the heels of the well-described effects of GLP-1's activation, and we can't say for sure that semaglutide can do something that GLP-1 *can't* do. However, because it reaches areas of the body that never encounter natural GLP-1 from the L-cells, we may see stronger effects. Quite simply, if GLP-1 were able to last longer in the body and reach those areas, it's most likely GLP-1 could accomplish everything that semaglutide does. On that note, it is a paradox when people argue that your body's naturally occurring GLP-1 has no significant effect.

Conversely, we can't say for sure that L-cell stimulation from undigested food can do something that semaglutide injected under the skin can't do. This is partly because GLP-1 from the L-cells accompanies other helpful hormones that affect appetite, blood sugar, inflammation, and sugar cravings (for example, GIP and PYY) as well as the quality of the gut barrier (GLP-2). Also, GLP-1 is released exactly where there are shortcuts to the aforementioned beta cells, as well as lots of nerves and immune cells, which can be affected by both the gut hormones and the compounds that well-nourished gut microbes share with us.

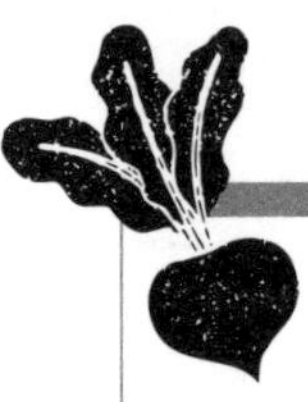

INVESTIGATING SOMETHING THAT DISAPPEARS LIKE DEW IN THE SUN

It is easy to study the effects of long-lasting hormone imitators in the body. On the other hand, it's difficult to study the effects of molecules that only survive for a few minutes. This is why it is perfectly normal to see an imbalance in the scientific rigor, which we should be aware of when discussing semaglutide and GLP-1. We have studied the body to understand GLP-1, and we have manufactured GLP-1 in a more long-lasting form than what the body itself creates.

Since we cannot directly compare the effects of GLP-1 and semaglutide, the burden of proof falls on all of us as we call for the use of the body's own capable biology in the struggle against obesity and the diseases resulting from it. Despite the seriousness of the matter, one that requires careful consideration, I'm certain we will succeed!

We have learned that treatment with GLP-1 medications has an amazing effect on appetite, weight, blood sugar, and food cravings. In addition, such treatment has an effect on addiction to and dependence on food, tobacco, alcohol, and drugs. On top of this—or as a consequence—effects on Alzheimer's disease, infertility, and a large number of cardiovascular diseases have been seen.

In short, GLP-1 apparently can counteract many of the negative results of a modern lifestyle characterized by too little movement and too much ultra-processed food. Considering how many friendly gut hormones we have, it is incredible that GLP-1 holds such great sway.

We can now ask ourselves whether the innate defects in the GLP-1 system can be important to many of us who get caught up in one or more of the negative health spirals characterized by the following:

- a decreased feeling of satiation

- high blood sugar

- insulin resistance

- addiction to sugar-rich ultra-processed food

- obesity, which increases insulin resistance, which increases poor appetite regulation and cravings for ultra-processed food

Could there be a direct correlation between difficulty feeling satiated and type 2 diabetes, obesity, and other illnesses? Are some people born with too little GLP-1 and thus feel an outsized addiction to food and become ashamed of the weight and diseases that follow? Or is it conceivable that we see this problem only in parts of the world where ultra-processed food has taken over, and hunger, satiation, and satisfaction have been replaced by food addiction?

If we look directly at GLP-1 alone, it does not appear to be the case that low levels of GLP-1 cause obesity. In a few studies, researchers have seen a connection between low GLP-1 levels and obesity, but most studies show no connection. If there is a correlation, it is unlikely to be insignificant. Conversely, well-nourished gut flora ensure the release of nutrients from your food to where the most L-cells are located, which can help satisfy you through the taste receptors in the small intestine, which are not connected to taste but to other nerve signals. This means that even if low GLP-1 does not *cause* obesity, encouraging your body to naturally produce more of it can help *reduce* obesity.

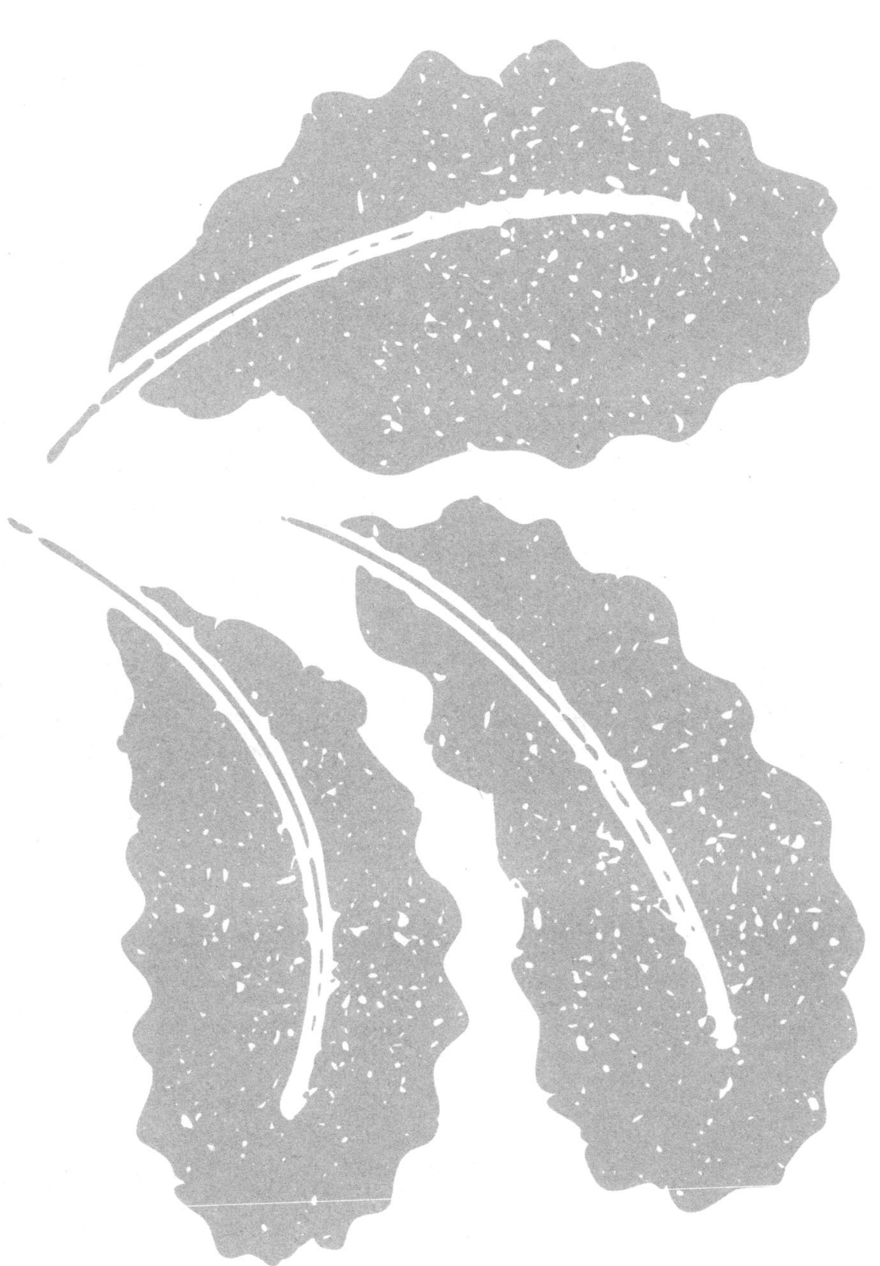

Chapter 11

When the switches stay off

In our busy and modern everyday life, we often steer toward quick, industrially processed meals. These foods are almost fully digested the moment they mix with the saliva in your mouth. As you know, that means the nutrients make only the short trip to your duodenum before you absorb them in a jiffy. On this express journey, nutrients do not have a chance to affect many L-cells, and sugar from the carbohydrates leads to a high blood sugar spike, which requires insulin. But because the food hasn't made it to the lower parts of the intestines yet, insulin has to manage without much help from its support rider, GLP-1.

This "new normal" is obviously exaggerated. What is not exaggerated is that most people connect obesity with eating too much food and burning too few calories. However, many studies—and the wider picture—indicate that this is a far too simplistic way of viewing health.

Perhaps we should flip this on its head and accept that, far too often, we provide too little nourishment to our gut microbes and L-cells, thus depriving them of the opportunity to boost our health. When we eat too much processed and ultra-processed, habit-forming food, designed to activate our innate more-wants-more instinct, our hungry gut flora are crying out for plant cells so that an active microbial community can be created for the benefit of our health.

The exaggerated new normal, as you know, does not only bypass GLP-1. It also bypasses a number of other metabolic hormones, which barely see the light of day when we eat lots of meals consisting of refined, carbohydrate-rich food. It will be exciting to see if replicas of several of the hormones suppressed by modern dietary habits—among them GIP, PYY, and glucagon—will follow in the footsteps of medications that mimic the effect of GLP-1 and spark genuine revolutions with significant consequences: reduced sales of ultra-processed food, reduced fuel consumption due to the reduced weight of passengers on planes, and—most importantly—far fewer diseases that go hand in hand with overeating, spiked blood sugar, and too much fat around the waist.

The food industry, which knows exactly what our primal brain is seeking, markets ultra-processed foods to us by labeling them as "low-sugar," "low-fat," "high-fiber," "high protein," and so on, shifting our focus away from the food's structure and composition to its ingredients. Our frustration at not losing weight when we follow these health claims makes us confused victims.

As these companies manipulate our addictive tendencies, profiting from our desire for instant gratification, we stop believing in ourselves and in our right to be healthy. All the while, social media, the country's leading news outlets, and the food and weight-loss industry shout about how difficult it is to lose weight, and that if you do lose weight, you should not expect to keep it off in the long run. Any belief in ourselves and the work our bodies can do is taken away from us, sacrificed upon the altar of capitalism and expert authority. This may sound like hyperbole, but it does not make the statement any less true. Remember how powerful you, your willpower, and your body are, and do not let anyone take that away from you. Your body is capable of more than you think, and you are smarter than you realize!

DESIRE AND ENJOYMENT

Desire and enjoyment are not the same thing, and I find myself wondering how many people who overeat habit-forming foods actually enjoy them. Do you? Once people are educated on the lasting harmful effects of a diet filled with ultra-processed foods, I can't imagine that many would actively choose to fill their stomachs with these products.

Imagine if natural GLP-1, which the body produces on its own when you avoid ultra-processed food and choose unprocessed, plant-rich food instead, could create more harmony between what you *crave* and what you *need*. Since the publication of my first book, *The Truth About Sugar,* I have traveled all around the world giving talks, teaching, taking part in debates and courses . . . the list goes on. Along the way, I've met thousands of people like you, and everywhere I go, I hear one story time after time.

A lot of good people tell me how they used to be addicted to the rush they got from ultra-processed food and have since dropped their addiction in favor of another vice. Now they simply cannot get enough of cabbage and other vegetables. The combination of satisfied gut microbes and stimulated L-cells ensures that these people are satisfied to a degree that Pepsi and pepperoni simply cannot compete with.

CLASH WITH THE CALORIE DICTATORSHIP

We once thought a calorie outside the body was the same as a calorie inside the body. Today, we know that some foods help us produce hormones that affect metabolism, appetite, the amount of brown fat in our bodies, and much more. We also know that the nutrients from unprocessed foods are shared with the millions of microorganisms in the gut, while we keep the entire calorie content from ultra-processed foods for ourselves. That does not mean calorie count is unimportant, but, to a large extent, it means calorie balance is not the only thing to consider.

Shame, guilt, overeating, an inability to maintain a healthy lifestyle in the long run, and lack of self-control are some of the negatives we associate with ourselves and others who are overweight. But let's turn that on its head in the name of lasting health.

Semaglutides, like Wegovy and Ozempic, and tirzepatides, like Zepbound, and other medications that mimic the effect of GLP-1 have made it clear to anyone who follows the news that obesity and overeating are complex issues with many dimensions. With the breakthrough effects of these medications, no one can continue to doubt that we have hormones that, to a large extent, affect our appetite, energy levels, metabolism, hunger levels, and food preferences.

Instead of turning us into passive injection users in one fell swoop, I propose starting a revolution with active, empowered, and well-informed people, with robust health and confidence in their own decisions. Both you and health professionals can bring about this revolution when armed with information about GLP-1. Healthcare professionals can pose questions to those looking for medical help with weight loss, such as the following:

1. Did you know that Wegovy (or Zepbound or others) mimics a hormone that you can ask your body to produce more of?

2. Would you like to learn more about this solution? It's free and leads to many other health benefits.

3. We used to place a lot of focus on how many calories we could consume when trying to lose weight. We've now discovered that ultra-processed food prevents us from empowering our body's own health mechanisms and turbocharging our metabolic engine. Do you want to know more about which foods have particularly good effects on your body's health mechanisms? A lot of people have benefited greatly from this strategy.

4. We now know that we have hormones that help us choose healthy foods and regulate our appetite. We feed these hormones when we eat plants, which the body digests in tandem with the thousands of friendly bacteria living in our gut. Do you want to know more about this exciting field, so we can see if you can benefit from this knowledge?

From many conversations with doctors, I know that this strategy works, because ultimately we humans want what's best for us. When it comes to our health, we want to take the bull by the horns, particularly when we've collaborated with our health-care provider to find the best solution for us!

Chapter 12

The other weight-loss hormones

As mentioned previously, GLP-1 is not the only weight-loss hormone in the field, but because of the amazing medications that have debuted on the market recently, we know far more about the effects of GLP-1 than we do about other weight-loss hormones. And we're only continuing to learn more.

As you read previously, a new group of medications is on the way, in which several weight-loss hormones have been combined into one drug. Our modern, inactive lifestyle, with the large proportion of ultra-processed food on the plate, prevents many different hormones from working properly, so—from a financial perspective—it makes a lot of sense to develop them all as medications. Particularly if our new normal will continue to consist of a large amount of ultra-processed food sprinkled with expensive medicine.

I will now tell you a little about the other natural weight-loss hormones.

GLUCAGON

You have encountered glucagon earlier in the book and may remember that the hormone is produced by the alpha cells in the pancreas. It functions as a counterweight to insulin in regulating blood sugar levels. While insulin lowers blood sugar by encouraging the intake of glucose in the body's cells, glucagon has the opposite effect: It raises blood sugar levels slightly by asking our liver to release glucose into the blood. Glucagon also has other effects on your metabolism.

1. **Elevated blood sugar:** When our blood sugar falls, the pancreas releases glucagon, which then signals to the liver that it should break down glycogen (the stored form of glucose) into glucose and release it into the bloodstream. This is particularly important between meals or during physical activity, when the body needs a steady injection of energy.

2. **Lipolysis:** Glucagon, under particular circumstances, also stimulates lipolysis, the process whereby fat cells break down triglycerides (fat) into free fatty acids, which can then be used as an energy source. This is also one of the mechanisms by which glucagon can contribute to weight loss. And this is where you get the entire argument why, ideally, we need glucagon to run its lap between all the insulin spikes. Because if we have insulin in the blood most of the day, glucagon never gets a chance to start burning fat. Researchers disagree about whether lipolysis occurs as a direct result of glucagon acting on the fat cells

or indirectly with the aid of our central nervous system. But for people who need to burn fat, it does not make much difference one way or the other if there is an intermediary in play.

3. **Ketogenesis:** Glucagon promotes ketogenesis, a process in which the liver transforms fatty acids into ketones, which can be used as a source of energy in periods with low carbohydrate intake or fasting. This process is central to ketogenic diets, which aim to promote fat burning.

4. **Appetite regulation:** There are indications that glucagon can affect our appetite. This happens as a direct result of the satiation-promoting ketones just mentioned, but it seems that glucagon can also affect appetite on its own.

By encouraging these four processes, glucagon can increase energy consumption and metabolism, even when resting. This can lead to a larger calorie deficit and subsequent weight loss, which is why it makes sense for the pharmaceutical industry to try to get glucagon on the market, because our modern lifestyle suppresses natural glucagon.

The weight-loss-boosting effects of glucagon should be understood in the context of its balance with insulin. Too much glucagon activity can lead to elevated blood sugar (hypoglycemia), which can be problematic for people with diabetes. So the balance between insulin and glucagon is crucial for healthy metabolic function. The two hormones have to interact like day and night, like hunger and satiation, like rest and exercise.

In summary, glucagon is a hormone that plays a central role in energy metabolism, particularly by promoting fat burning and increasing blood sugar in periods with energy demands.

GIP

GIP is another hormone that the pharmaceutical industry is focusing on for the treatment of obesity. Like GLP-1, GIP has an impact on the insulin deliveries of the beta cells, and there are indications that it also affects brown fat tissue.

GIP is delivered from some GLP-1-containing L-cells but also from other enteroendocrine cells in the digestive system, namely the K-cells. Unlike the L-cells, these are densely situated in the upper part of the duodenum, while there are fewer K-cells as we move further down the intestine.

Unlike GLP-1, GIP does not seem to have a major effect on its own, while there is much to indicate that the hormone can reinforce the effects of GLP-1. GLP-1 and GIP activity are combined in tirzepatide medications such as Zepbound.

AMYLIN

Amylin is a hormone secreted by the pancreas along with insulin. The hormone has several functions that contribute to weight regulation:

1. **Appetite regulation:** Amylin affects the brain, particularly areas like the hypothalamus, which is responsible for appetite adjustment. When amylin is secreted after a meal, it signals to the brain that the body is full, which reduces the hunger sensation and affects the amount of

food you put on your plate. This appetite-suppressing effect can help reduce your calorie intake, which is definitely not without significance for losing weight.

2. **Delayed gastric emptying:** Amylin slows the emptying of the stomach (like GLP-1), meaning the food stays in the stomach longer. This leads to a prolonged feeling of satiation, which can also contribute to reducing the frequency of meals and reducing the number of calories consumed.

3. **Inhibition of glucagon secretion:** Amylin fine-tunes the release of glucagon, which normally increases blood sugar by stimulating the liver's release of glucose. By inhibiting glucagon, amylin can help prevent spikes in blood sugar after meals, which can reduce the urge to eat and can help with weight loss.

PYY

Peptide YY (PYY) is a hormone that is primarily produced and released in the gut's L-cells along with GLP-1. PYY also plays an important role in the regulation of appetite and digestive processes.

1. **Appetite regulation:** PYY works in the brain's hypothalamus, where it inhibits another peptide, neuropeptide Y (NPY). It is a powerful appetite-stimulating peptide. By inhibiting NPY, PYY reduces the appetite, which of course leads to reduced food intake.

2. **Delayed gastric emptying:** Like GLP-1 and amylin, PYY slows the emptying of the stomach. This contributes to an extended feeling of fullness after meals, which also helps to reduce your calorie intake.

3. **Adjustment of the pancreas:** PYY can inhibit the discharge of digestive enzymes and bile acids, slowing the digestion and absorption of nutrients. In principle, this can ensure that even more food remnants reach the areas of the gut where there are lots of L-cells, so we gain even more benefit from GLP-1, GIP, and yes, PYY itself, all working in health synergy.

4. **Adjustment of sugar cravings:** Some research indicates that PYY can reduce your cravings for sugar. PYY's role in appetite regulation and specifically in reducing cravings for sweet and calorie-rich foods has been the subject of many studies. There is much to indicate that PYY affects the brain's reward system, which plays a central role when it comes to sugar cravings. By counteracting the rewarding effects of sugary foods, PYY can reduce the cravings that often drive us to eat sugar, even when we're not hungry. It has been proven that higher levels of PYY after a meal are connected with lower cravings for sugary foods.

GLP-2

GLP-2 is a cousin of GLP-1, and they are both put into circulation by the L-cells in the gut. Although GLP-2 does not belong to the category of weight-loss hormones, it deserves to be honored for all the good work it does for your health. GLP-2 has at least two important effects—the strengthening of the gut's mucous membrane and the strengthening of your bones. Without going further into GLP-2 here, I would like to remind you that an inflamed, leaky gut and osteoporosis are two serious additional conditions proven to be linked to a diet filled with ultra-processed foods.

Chapter 13

The world requires both medicine and knowledge

It's not up to me to decide whether you should consider medication or try to activate more GLP-1 through lifestyle changes. That decision is entirely up to you but should be made after a healthy conversation with your doctor, because the question is very individual, and there are already enough armchair professionals out there whose opinions may not always be well-informed.

But I hear from family physicians and registered nurses that a perfectly harmless conversation about natural GLP-1 has led to plenty of good weight-loss and disease-remission outcomes. While obesity can be difficult to discuss, a conversation about natural weight-loss hormones can be a relief to share with others.

In a knowledge-based society, on the other hand, we can't just accept that so many people believe medication is the only solution to the issue of high blood sugar and weight, when small lifestyle changes and a diet rich in vegetables (rather than ultra-processed products) can in many instances be a key part of the solution.

WHAT SHOULD I DO–
AND WHAT SHOULD I KNOW?

I've explained that the body produces its own GLP-1, that GLP-1 is accompanied by other gut hormones, and that the body breaks down GLP-1 quickly if it escapes and enters the bloodstream. You also know that surgical shortcuts in your intestines, brought about by bariatric surgery, will cause your body to produce far more GLP-1—most likely because it sends more undigested food to the areas that have the highest densities of cells that release GLP-1.

You also get more unprocessed food to the L-cells when you eat food that is not predigested by the food industry, and earlier in the book we determined what is processed and what is unprocessed, and why it is so important to understand what you're putting in your body.

With all these factors affecting GLP-1, it is surely no surprise that there is no single well-documented lifestyle that will get your body to produce the optimal amount of GLP-1 for the way you live—although I will venture to give my best suggestion shortly.

But with our modern reality, more than half of our disease burden is linked to obesity, blood sugar, inflammation, and the consequences arising from them. And particularly for these kinds of conditions, individual empowerment is an important factor. If we use ourselves as resources in this, we can slow the development and severity of type 2 diabetes, elevated blood pressure, cardiovascular diseases, cancers, autoimmune diseases, and much, much more.

The question here is whether the quick instructions and the wagging finger have failed, while biological knowledge and positive incentives toward joint responsibility and the importance of individual choice will pay off in the long run. That is what I am advocating.

Individual choice and a commitment to health are played down in clinical studies of high scientific quality to avoid so-called bias. But the reality of creating a healthier world has to be founded on knowledge, commitment, empowerment, and responsibility, because it is influence, empowerment, and freedom that promote good health and quality of life.

Before you put this book down, I would like to summarize how I propose you structure your day if you want a body that works toward healthy insulin sensitivity, thriving gut flora, L-cells that are allowed to excel at what they do best, and a healthy body weight. If you test out the following methods, I'm confident you can experience significant weight loss from the outset, and your blood sugar can be normalized in only a few days or weeks. The effect of being uncompromising in keeping stable blood sugar and pampering your gut flora is in many ways similar to the effect of the surgeries described at the beginning of this book. For some, this uncompromisingly stable–blood sugar and gut-flora-pampering lifestyle seems practically miraculous, which is why many are surprised they did not receive this advice a long time ago. But you have to promise me two things:

1. Include your doctor in your considerations if you're going to scale back on medication (for example, for type 2 diabetes, high blood pressure, or pain) when you change your relationship to food.

2. If you have nice people around you who you think can benefit from the knowledge in this book, refrain from telling them what they can or should do. Instead, encourage them to discover the same fascination with the body's biology that I hope you have found in this book. When it comes to food, nitpicking what people should or shouldn't eat simply doesn't work. And it may be one of the biggest reasons why most diets fail in the long run. Success requires personal ownership and responsibility along with wisdom, support, and discipline.

So when you read the following, I encourage you to focus on what's on your own plate and consider yourself an empowered person who takes responsibility through knowledge.

It's easier to change your own choices than to change the world.

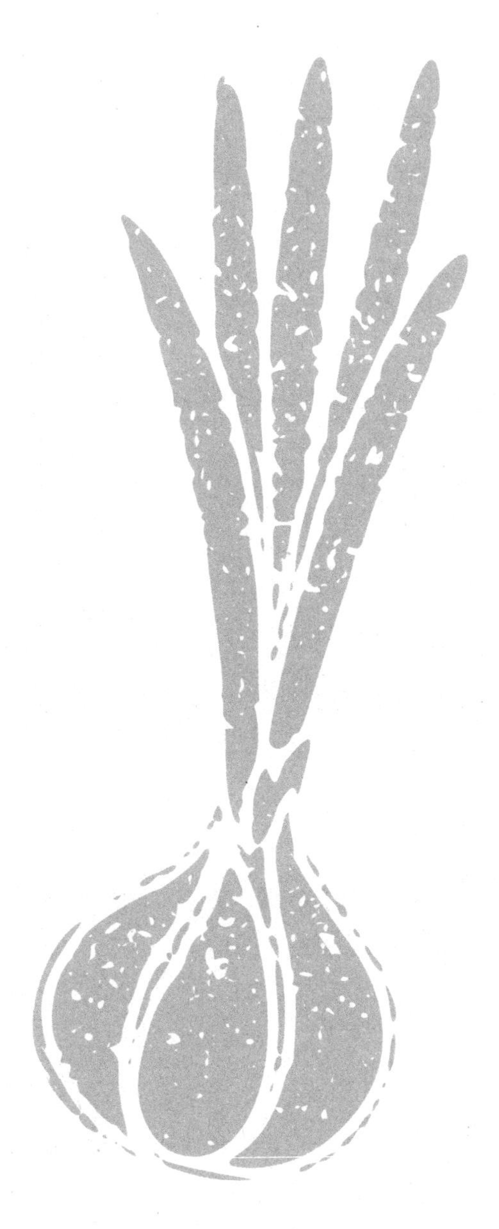

Chapter 14

This is how you create your healthy body

I have tried to impart a lot of my knowledge about the weight-loss hormone GLP-1, insulin resistance, blood sugar, inflammation, and the importance of a synergy with your gut flora. In addition to your new knowledge, you will now find my best recipe for an optimal balance between all of these things. Not because I necessarily believe you have to live that way for your entire life, but because it should be your *default* setting, which you can deviate from according to your wants, needs, and choices.

And then I would venture to assert that all adults, for longer or shorter periods each year, will benefit from taking note of what that lifestyle does to your body. We are talking about five things:

- unprocessed food

- only three meals every day

- exercise

- sleep

- exposure to cold

THE PERFECT PLATE

As you know, eating whole plant cells and unprocessed food is the best way to achieve stable blood sugar, well-fed gut flora, and a life where L-cells are exposed to the nutrients and flavor and color compounds that release GLP-1 and the other intestinal hormones that contribute to your well-being. At the same time, what you choose to eat affects how quickly nutrients are absorbed, which can then lead to either steady blood sugar or significant fluctuations. So what should you put on your plate?

My books always take an uncompromising starting point, giving you the chance to experience the full health benefits. When you have lived an uncompromising week or two, you can consider whether to maintain your new routine or reintroduce a few favorite meals or energy sources to get you through the week or on special occasions.

Everything that goes on your plate during an uncompromising week is unprocessed and low in carbohydrates, and you can get much more inspiration in the section about ultra-processed and unprocessed foods. In the illustration on page 139, the uncompromising week should contain only foods from the lower-left box—and they should be put together based on your favorite dishes, so the plate is constructed as you see in the illustration on the right.

If you use online resources to find recipes, make sure all ingredients appear in the lower-left box. If they don't, you can make simple swaps or omissions based on your knowledge of the foods that activate your intrinsic health.

	UNPROCESSED	PROCESSED
HIGH CARB	• Fruit • Good-quality, seeded rye bread • Rice • Grains, oats, corn, rye, and so on • Lentils and pulses with a high content of accessible carbohydrates • Potatoes	• Ice cream, candy, soda, and cake • Bread containing refined grain and/or preservatives • Many types of yogurt containing fruit • Breakfast cereals • Many plant drinks and dairy alternatives
LOW CARB	• Cabbage and other coarse vegetables • All vegetables and herbs • Pulses and lentils rich in easily digestible carbohydrates • Cheese, milk, butter, skyr, kefir, and plain Greek yogurt • Nuts, almonds, and seeds • Eggs, meat, fish, and shellfish • Oils, avocado, and other fats • Tempeh, tofu, yeast flakes, and pure protein products	• Highly refined breads (such as gluten-free bread) • Food with added potato, corn, or wheat flour • Many meat substitutes • Seitan • Some plant-based drinks, vegan creamers, and plant-based yogurt
	UNPROCESSED	PROCESSED

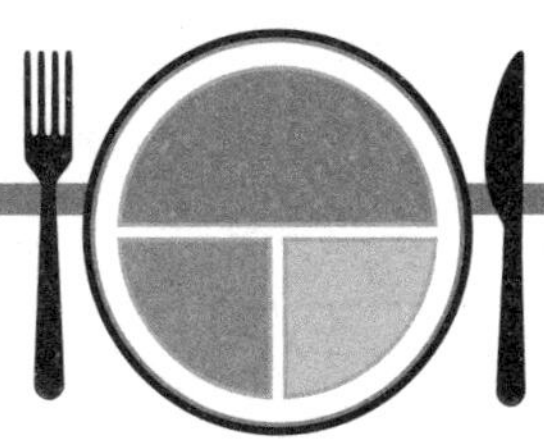

THE UNCOMPROMISING STARTING POINT IS A PLATE MODEL CONSISTING OF THE FOLLOWING:

25 PERCENT CABBAGE AND OTHER COARSE VEGETABLES

These include cabbage, broccoli, cauliflower, kale, sprouts, lettuce, Brussels sprouts, spinach, and other coarse vegetables. It's okay to fry, bake, grill, boil, blend, freeze, or whatever else you can think of. Of course, you should not add sugar or flour, but you can certainly include plenty of herbs, chiles, and other spices, as well as good fats.

50 PERCENT VEGETABLES

This part of the plate can contain vegetables from anywhere in the world, including cucumber, squash, tomato, eggplant, mushrooms, peas, beans, celeriac, parsnip, and all the cabbages and coarse vegetables from the preceding section. You can continue the list yourself.

25 PERCENT GOOD FAT AND PROTEIN SOURCES

These include nuts, almonds, seeds, avocados, good-quality tofu, high-protein lentils and beans, and healthy oils. You can also eat eggs, skyr, kefir, natural yogurt (that is, nothing with added sugar), cheese, butter, good-quality meat, and shellfish.

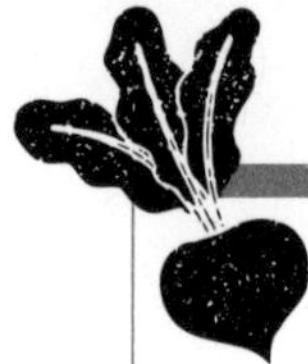

BIOLOGIC SQUARES–
YOUR PERSONAL GPS

On the bottom axis, we divide foods into unprocessed and processed, corresponding to the whole plant cells and refined nutrient molecules from the illustration on page 138.

On the other axis, we divide foods into those with a low carbohydrate content and those with a high carbohydrate content. Remember that you can get the nutrients you need without having to experience blood sugar spikes.

In the lower-left square, you can find all the nutrients you need. Here you will also find all the good sources of fat and protein–both for those who eat everything and for those who enjoy a vegetarian or vegan diet. All food in the lower-left square is low in carbohydrates. At the same time, your food is shared with your gut bacteria, which distributes the nutrients to your L-cells.

Indulgences from the upper-right square are guaranteed to lead to blood sugar spikes, while the two lighter squares can cause blood sugar spikes in insulin-resistant people, but rarely in people with high insulin sensitivity.

Obviously, it is all a matter of quantity. But you know all about that. The more consistently you stick to foods in the lower-left quadrant, the better your intestinal flora and your weight-loss hormones can help guide you onto the right path, so you are not carrying all the responsibility alone. And the further you are from your goal, the more uncompromising you will have to be.

You may be surprised that rice, bread, and potatoes are not found in the lower-left part of the biologic squares. I understand your amazement, because it is often recommended that you eat whole grains if you want to maintain a healthy lifestyle. You will not receive that recommendation from me. This is because all grains are high in carbohydrates and, particularly during your uncompromising week, you have to maintain relatively stable blood sugar, meaning you need little insulin to regain your high insulin sensitivity.

However, many people can certainly add potatoes, oats, and rye bread to their meal if they need a little more energy than they get from vegetables alone. But again, my recommendation is that you first try to manage without them if you are an adult in search of health and weight balance.

If you swear by whole grains (which are obviously a thousand times better than bread made from ultra-refined white flour, which barely reaches the first bend of your intestines), you should be cautious. Read the labeling and check how much sugar and refined flour has actually been added. Many whole-grain products contain only 10 percent whole grain.

To spell it out for you, if you're insulin-sensitive, you can certainly add a little fruit, whole-grain bread, rice, and occasional snacks if you feel like it. If you're insulin-resistant and struggling with unwanted weight, like more than 50 percent of the population, you should stay away from refined and carbohydrate-rich foods. The same applies if you want to regain insulin sensitivity, appetite regulation, weight regulation, and the ability to feel satiated.

ONLY THREE MAIN MEALS A DAY

Breaks between meals create the best insulin sensitivity, bring glucagon into play, and reduce the risk of your own hormones from the stomach preventing the L-cells from producing GLP-1. So my recommendation is to eat three solid meals a day instead of fasting for parts of the day or several days. But you can play with this plan and adjust it as it suits you.

The fact is, if you stick to unprocessed food, then everything works. Everything! Ultimately, it is the addiction to ultra-processed foods that keeps us trapped as low-energy food junkies in the iron grip of the food industry.

EXERCISE—USE YOUR MUSCLES

I also mentioned that exercise may be able to trigger the release of the neurotransmitter CGRP, which—if it reaches the L-cells—can ensure that even more GLP-1 is released. This is a good thing.

But exercise can do much more than that. Exercise can ensure that you burn calories, and it can make sure you maintain your muscle mass. At the same time, exercising your muscles makes you hypersensitive to insulin, so the muscles—a key player in maintaining stable blood sugar—absorb excess sugar from the blood in a flash, ensuring healthy insulin sensitivity.

People swear by different forms of exercise, but the main thing is to get *some* form of exercise. I recommend that you move your body for at least half an hour every day and that you use every opportunity during the day to briefly get your pulse up by having a pulse snack or exercise snack instead of a traditional snack. How you temporarily raise your pulse (I recommend at least four times a day) is entirely up to you. Go for a run, take a little stroll, use the stairs instead of the elevator, do fifteen jumping squats, plank for one minute, or wall-sit for two minutes. Everything works. Don't overcomplicate things. Do it in secret or tempt others to join you. Just do it.

SLEEP

Getting seven to nine hours of sleep every night boosts your insulin sensitivity and the healthy interaction between insulin and glucagon, which operate as security guards for your energy storage. Sleep repairs a lot of the processes in your body, and because you're (most likely) not eating while you sleep, you're also giving your body several hours of proper fasting. This is why sleep presents you with a unique opportunity to put glucagon and fat burning to work during the night.

If you get a good night's sleep, you wake up the next day far more insulin-sensitive. If you have stable blood sugar tomorrow, there is a good chance you will also have it the following day.

Remember that high blood sugar can activate your immune system by randomly attaching sugar to your own proteins, causing your immune system to react to those proteins. You can clean up that mess by going to sleep with stable blood sugar.

COLD

This is the first of my books where I recommend exposing your body to shifts in temperature. Temperature fluctuations experienced while winter bathing or taking cold showers cause the body to burn extra calories and give you a chance to create brown fat, which you can put to good use to keep warm.

Ultra-processed food and all the modes of transport that do not require muscular activity hold an enormous responsibility for the current obesity and disease epidemics, but could maintaining a comfortable seventy degrees indoors—in summer and winter—also share some of the blame?

Experiment! Play a little with the extremes. Take a cold dip in the sea or the lake or turn on the cold water for a moment when you have your morning shower. Move around to get warm afterward. And take heed of the old advice from your grandmother about keeping the temperature in your bedroom a little lower.

And remember—a comfortable life is not necessarily the same as a good and happy life. Life without a little struggle is not much of a life. The best moments are enjoyed when you've had to fight for them a little.

Conclusion
Your health is in your hands

I hope you have enjoyed learning all about the body's own weight-loss hormones—including the digressions we've taken along the way. There are so many ways to pursue a healthy life and a healthy weight these days. Scientific research has developed some truly life-changing medications that can help those who struggle with their weight, and these are significant advancements we should celebrate.

As amazing as these medications are for many, particularly in the ways they mimic and enhance the incredible cascade of effects that real food triggers in our bodies, we must also acknowledge they can be cost-prohibitive to some, and not everyone reacts well to them. This is why I wrote this book: to share knowledge and give people access to education about your body's own impressive resources and abilities. I want everyone to have the tools they need to make the best decisions, along with their healthcare provider, for themselves. I cannot tolerate the fact that it is easier to get a prescription than it is to access basic biological knowledge about this competent body of yours!

My wish for you is a long and healthy life with all the freedom to make your own choices. And lots of vegetables! Always lots of vegetables.

Thank you

To everyone at Gyldendal and Ten Speed Press for your work and support on this book.

A special thank-you to editor Henriette Maria Meier-Jensen, who convinced me to write this book; to the head of publishing, Mette Korsgaard; and to editor Mikkel Fønsskov for taking over in the final phase when Henriette sought new challenges. Writing books with all of you is never dull.

To Søren Frandsen, for generously sharing your linguistic talent in my books.

To Maria Bramsen, for making the book exceptionally beautiful and full of illustrations.

To Professor Jens Juul Holst, for your admirable and vital research into GLP-1 and for how you share your insights with the world.

A special thank-you to all of my amazing former colleagues at Novo Nordisk for their exciting scientific discussions about GLP-1, obesity, and diabetes and for the nuanced conversations about all the dilemmas in the treatment of type 2 diabetes and obesity.

And the biggest thank-you of all goes to the best family in the world, for their support (and loving headshakes) on another book project.

Finally, a heartfelt thanks to you, my new or loyal reader, for your interest in how you can let your body do the work.

References

The following section contains references to the works and articles used as sources and background material in the preparation of this book. The references are grouped by topic, and you will find articles in Danish at www.videnskab.dk as well as scientific and peer-reviewed research articles in English. I also recommend a number of books for further reading on related topics.

THE REGULATION OF GLP-1 BY THE BODY AND BY FOOD

Bodnaruc, A. M., Prud'homme, D., Blanchet, R., & Giroux, I. (2016). Nutritional modulation of endogenous glucagon-like peptide-1 secretion: a review. *Nutrition & Metabolism*, 13, 92.

Brubaker, P. L., & Anini, Y. (2003). Direct and indirect mechanisms regulating secretion of glucagon-like peptide-1 and glucagon-like peptide-2. *Canadian Journal of Physiology and Pharmacology*, 81(11), 1005–1012.

Domínguez Avila, J. A., Rodrigo García, J., González Aguilar, G. A., & de la Rosa, L. A. (2017). The antidiabetic mechanisms of polyphenols related to increased glucagon-like peptide-1 (GLP1) and insulin signaling. *Molecules* (Basel, Switzerland), 22(6), 903.

Dubé, P. E., & Brubaker, P. L. (2004). Nutrient, neural and endocrine control of glucagon-like peptide secretion. *Hormone and Metabolic Research*, 36(11/12), 755–760.

Gribble, F. M., & Reimann, F. (2016). Enteroendocrine cells: chemosensors in the intestinal epithelium. *Annual Review of Physiology*, 78(1), 277–299.

Holst, J. J. (2007). The physiology of glucagon-like peptide 1. *Physiological Reviews, 87*(4), 1409–1439.

Holst, J. J. (2019). The incretin system in healthy humans: the role of GIP and GLP-1. *Metabolism, Clinical and Experimental, 96,* 46–55.

Holst, J. J. (2024). GLP-1 physiology in obesity and development of incretin-based drugs for chronic weight management. *Nature Metabolism, 6*(10), 1866–1885.

Huber, H., Schieren, A., Holst, J. J., & Simon, M. C. (2024). Dietary impact on fasting and stimulated GLP-1 secretion in different metabolic conditions—a narrative review. *American Journal of Clinical Nutrition,* 119(3), 599–627.

Hunt, J. E., Hartmann, B., Schoonjans, K., Holst, J. J., & Kissow, H. (2021). Dietary fiber is essential to maintain intestinal size, L-cell secretion, and intestinal integrity in mice. *Frontiers in Endocrinology* (Lausanne), 12, 640602.

Jeppesen, P. B., Dorner, A., Yue, Y., Poulsen, N., Andersen, S. K., Aalykke, F. B., & Lambert, M. N. T. (2024). Beneficial effects of a freeze-dried kale bar on type 2 diabetes patients: a randomized, double-blinded, placebo-controlled clinical trial. *Nutrients,* 16(21), 3641.

Kuhre, R. E., Deacon, C. F., Holst, J. J., & Petersen, N. (2021). What is an L-cell and how do we study the secretory mechanisms of the L-cell? *Frontiers in Endocrinology* (Lausanne), 12, 694284.

Nilsson, C., Hansen, T. K., Rosenquist, C., Hartmann, B., Kodra, J. T., Lau, J. F., Clausen, T. R., Raun, K., & Sams, A. (2016). Long-acting analogue of the calcitonin gene-related peptide induces positive metabolic effects and secretion of the glucagon-like peptide-1. *European Journal of Pharmacology,* 773, 24–31.

Ortega-Hernández, E., Antunes-Ricardo, M., & Jacobo-Velázquez, D. A. (2021). Improving the health-benefits of kales (Brassica oleracea L. var. acephala DC) through the application of controlled abiotic stresses: a review. *Plants* (Basel, Switzerland), 10(12), 2629.

Spreckley, E., & Murphy, K. G. (2015). The L-cell in nutritional sensing and the regulation of appetite. *Frontiers in Nutrition* (Lausanne), 2, 23.

Steinert, R. E., Feinle-Bisset, C., Asarian, L., Horowitz, M., Beglinger, C., & Geary, N. (2017). Ghrelin, CCK, GLP-1, and PYY (3–36): secretory controls and physiological roles in eating and glycemia in health, obesity, and after RYGB. *Physiological Reviews*, 97(1), 411–463.

Wang, Q., Lin, H., Shen, C., Zhang, M., Wang, X., Yuan, M., Yuan, M., Jia, S., Cao, Z., Wu, C., Chen, B., Gao, A., Bi, Y., Ning, G., Wang, W., Wang, J., & Liu, R. (2023). Gut microbiota regulates postprandial GLP-1 response via ileal bile acid-TGR5 signaling. *Gut Microbes*, 15(2), 2274124.

ULTRA-PROCESSED FOOD

Lane, M. M., Gamage, E., Du, S., Ashtree, D. N., McGuinness, A. J., Gauci, S., Baker, P., Lawrence, M., Rebholz, C. M., Srour, B., Touvier, M., Jacka, F. N., O'Neil, A., Segasby, T., & Marx, W. (2024). Ultra-processed food exposure and adverse health outcomes: umbrella review of epidemiological meta-analyses. *BMJ* (Online), 28:384, e077310.

Martínez Steele, E., Juul, F., Neri, D., Rauber, F., & Monteiro, C. A. (2019). Dietary share of ultra-processed foods and metabolic syndrome in the US adult population. *Preventive Medicine*, 125, 40–48.

Monteiro, C. A., Cannon, G., Levy, R. B., Moubarac, J.-C., Louzada, M. L., Rauber, F., Khandpur, N., Cediel, G., Neri, D., Martinez-Steele, E., Baraldi, L. G., & Jaime, P. C. (2019). Ultra-processed foods: what they are and how to identify them. *Public Health Nutrition*, 22(5), 936–941.

van Tulleken, C. (2023). *Ultra-Processed People.* Penguin (Cornerstone).

Monteiro, C. A., Moubarac, J.-C., Levy, R. B., Canella, D. S., Louzada, M. L. da C., & Cannon, G. (2018). Household availability of ultra-processed foods and obesity in nineteen European countries. *Public Health Nutrition*, 21(1), 18–26.

Rico-Campà, A., Martínez-González, M. A., Alvarez-Alvarez, I., Mendonça, R. de D., de la Fuente-Arrillaga, C., Gómez-Donoso, C., & Bes-Rastrollo, M. (2019). Association between consumption of ultra-processed foods and all cause mortality: SUN prospective cohort study. *BMJ* (Online), 29:365, l949.

WEB

Blomhoff, R. (2023). Nordic nutrition recommendations 2023: integrating environmental aspects. New edition. Nordic Council of Ministers/Nordisk Ministerråd. https://pub.norden.org/nord2023-003/introduction.html.

Spilde, I. (2024) Kæmpe studie kobler ultraforarbejdet mad til mange sygdomme—men hvad betyder det? Videnskab DK/Videnskab.dk.

https://videnskab.dk/krop-sundhed/kaempe-studie-kobler-ultraforarbej -det-mad-til-mange-sygdomme-men-hvad-betyder-det/.

Woods, J., Lawrence, M., Machado, P. & Dickie, S. (2023). Sådan spotter du ultraforarbejdede fødevarer. Videnskab DK/Videnskab.dk.

https://videnskab.dk/krop-sundhed/8-helt-almindelige-foedevarer-som -er-ultraforarbejdede-uden-du-ved-det/.

GLP-1 AND ITS RECEPTOR, DEGRADATION, AND MORE

Deacon, C. F., Pridal, L., Klarskov, L., Olesen, M., & Holst, J. J. (1996). Glucagon-like peptide 1 undergoes differential tissue-specific metabolism in the anesthetized pig. *American Journal of Physiology: Endocrinology and Metabolism*, 271(3), E458–E464.

Hui, H., Farilla, L., Merkel, P., & Perfetti, R. (2002). The short half-life of glucagon-like peptide-1 in plasma does not reflect its long-lasting beneficial effects. *European Journal of Endocrinology*, 146(6), 863–869.

Meier, J. J., Nauck, M. A., Kranz, D., Holst, J. J., Deacon, C. F., Gaeckler, D., Schmidt, W. E., & Gallwitz, B. (2004). Secretion, degradation, and elimination of glucagon-like peptide 1 and gastric inhibitory polypeptide in patients with chronic renal insufficiency and healthy control subjects. *Diabetes* (New York), 53(3), 654–662.

Müller, T. D., Finan, B., Bloom, S. R., D'Alessio, D., Drucker, D. J., Flatt, P. R., Fritsche, A., Gribble, F., Grill, H. J., Habener, J. F., Holst, J. J., Langhans, W., Meier, J. J., Nauck, M. A., Perez-Tilve, D., Pocai, A., Reimann, F., Sandoval, D. A., Schwartz, T. W., . . . & Tschöp, M. H. (2019). Glucagon-like peptide 1 (GLP-1). *Molecular Metabolism* (Germany), 30, 72–130.

Tomas, A., Jones, B., & Leech, C. (2020). New insights into beta-cell GLP-1 receptor and cAMP signaling. *Journal of Molecular Biology*, 432(5), 1347–1366.

OZEMPIC AND WEGOVY

Ozempic (information for healthcare personnel). https://pro.medicin.dk/ Medicin/Praeparater/8714.

Wegovy FlexTouch (information for healthcare personnel). https://min
.medicin.dk/Medicin/Praeparater/10247.

THE EFFECTS OF GLP-1

Drucker, D. J. (2018). Mechanisms of action and therapeutic application of glucagon-like peptide-1. *Cell Metabolism, 27*(4), 740–756.

Hropot, T., Herman, R., Janez, A., Lezaic, L., & Jensterle, M. (2023). Brown adipose tissue: a new potential target for glucagon-like peptide 1 receptor agonists in the treatment of obesity. *International Journal of Molecular Sciences,* 11:24(10), 8592.

López-Ferreras, L., Richard, J. E., Noble, E. E., Eerola, K., Anderberg, R. H., Olandersson, K., Taing, L., Kanoski, S. E., Hayes, M. R., & Skibicka, K. P. (2018). Lateral hypothalamic GLP-1 receptors are critical for the control of food reinforcement, ingestive behavior and body weight. *Molecular Psychiatry, 23*(5), 1157–1168.

Madsbad, S., & Holst, J. J. (2023). Cardiovascular effects of incretins: focus on glucagon-like peptide-1 receptor agonists. *Cardiovascular Research, 119*(4), 886–904.

A LITTLE ABOUT BROWN FAT—THOUGH OPINIONS DIFFER AMONG SCIENTISTS AROUND THE WORLD

Beiroa, D., Imbernon, M., Gallego, R., Senra, A., Herranz, D., Villarroya, F., Serrano, M., Fernø, J., Salvador, J., Escalada, J., Dieguez, C., Lopez, M., Frühbeck, G., & Nogueiras, R. (2014). GLP-1 agonism stimulates brown adipose tissue thermogenesis and browning through hypothalamic AMPK. *Diabetes* (New York), 63(10), 3346–3358.

Hachemi, I., & U-Din, M. (2023). Brown adipose tissue: activation and metabolism in humans. *Endocrinology and Metabolism* (Seoul), 38(2), 214–222.

Locie, S. H., Heppner, K. M., Rahmouni, K., Oldfield, B. J., Tschöp, M. H., Perez-Tilve, D., Chaudhary, N., Chabenne, J. R., Morgan, D. A., Veyrat-Durebex, C., Ananthakrishnan, G., Rohner-Jeanrenaud, F., Drucker, D. J., & Dimarchi, R. (2012). Direct control of brown adipose tissue thermogenesis by central nervous system glucagon-like peptide-1 receptor signaling. *Diabetes* (New York), 61(11), 2753–2762.

Panchal, S. K., Bliss, E., & Brown, L. (2018). Capsaicin in metabolic syndrome. *Nutrients,* 17:10(5), 630.

WEB

Svennevig, B. (2024). Kan det brune fedt hjælpe os i kampen mod fedme? Syddansk Universitet/SDU.dk. https://www.sdu.dk/da/om-sdu/ fakulteterne/naturvidenskab/nyhe-der-2024/brown-fat-nature -metabolism.

OBESITY OPERATIONS AFFECTING GLP-1

DePaula, A. L., Macedo, A. L. V., Rassi, N., Vencio, S., Machado, C. A., Mota, B. R., Silva, L. Q., Halpern, A., & Schraibman, V. (2008). Laparoscopic treatment of metabolic syndrome in patients with type 2 diabetes mellitus. *Surgical Endoscopy,* 22(12), 2670–2678.

Dirksen, C., Damgaard, M., Bojsen-Møller, K. N., Jørgensen, N. B., Kielgast, U., Jacobsen, S. H., Naver, L. S., Worm, D., Holst, J. J., Madsbad, S., Hansen, D. L., & Madsen, J. L. (2013). Fast pouch emptying, delayed small intestinal transit, and exaggerated gut hormone responses after Roux-en-Y gastric bypass. *Neurogastroenterology and Motility,* 25(4), 255–346.

Grueneberger, J. M., Fritz, T., Zhou, C., Meyer, S., Karcz-Socha, I., Sawczyn, T., Stygar, D., Goos, M., Hopt, U. T., & Küsters, S. (2013). Long segment ileal transposition leads to early amelioration of glucose control in the diabetic obese Zucker rat. *Wideochirurgia i Inne Techniki Mało Inwazyjne,* 8(2), 130–138.

Hindsø, M., Bojsen-Møller, K. N., Kristiansen, V. B., Holst, J. J., van Hall, G., & Madsbad, S. (2022). Early effects of Roux-en-Y gastric bypass on dietary fatty acid absorption and metabolism in people with obesity and normal glucose tolerance. *International Journal of Obesity,* 46(7), 1359–1365.

Kindel, T. L., Yoder, S. M., Seeley, R. J., D'Alessio, D. A., & Tso, P. (2009). Duodenal-jejunal exclusion improves glucose tolerance in the diabetic, goto-kakizaki rat by a GLP-1 receptor-mediated mechanism. *Journal of Gastrointestinal Surgery,* 13(10), 1762–1772.

Martinussen, C., Bojsen-Møller, K. N., Dirksen, C., Svane, M. S., Kristiansen, V. B., Hartmann, B., Holst, J. J., & Madsbad, S. (2019).

Augmented GLP-1 secretion as seen after gastric bypass may be obtained by delaying carbohydrate digestion. *Journal of Clinical Endocrinology and Metabolism, 104*(8), 3233–3244.

Odstrcil, E. A., Martinez, J. G., Santa Ana, C. A., Xue, B., Schneider, R. E., Steffer, K. J., Porter, J. L., Asplin, J., Kuhn, J. A., & Fordtran, J. S. (2010). The contribution of malabsorption to the reduction in net energy absorption after long-limb Roux-en-Y gastric bypass. *American Journal of Clinical Nutrition, 92*(4), 704–713.

Patriti, A., Facchiano, E., Annetti, C., Aisa, M. C., Galli, F., Fanelli, C., & Donini, A. (2005). Early improvement of glucose tolerance after ileal transposition in a non-obese type 2 diabetes rat model. *Obesity Surgery, 15*(9), 1258–1264.

Schauer, P. R., Bhatt, D. L., Kirwan, J. P., Wolski, K., Aminian, A., Brethauer, S. A., Navaneethan, S. D., Singh, R. P., Pothier, C. E., Nissen, S. E., & Kashyap, S. R. (2017). Bariatric surgery versus intensive medical therapy for diabetes—5-year outcomes. *New England Journal of Medicine, 376*(7), 641–651.

Tan, T., Behary, P., Tharakan, G., Minnion, J., Al-Najim, W., Albrechtsen, N. J. W., Holst, J. J., & Bloom, S. R. (2017). The effect of a subcutaneous infusion of GLP-1, OXM, and PYY on energy intake and expenditure in obese volunteers. *Journal of Clinical Endocrinology and Metabolism, 102*(7), 2364–2372.

SOME MUSCLES DO MORE FOR YOUR METABOLIC HEALTH THAN OTHERS

Hamilton, M. T., Hamilton, D. G., & Zderic, T. W. (2022). A potent physiological method to magnify and sustain soleus oxidative metabolism improves glucose and lipid regulation. *iScience, 25*(9), 104869.

ABOUT THE OTHER WEIGHT-LOSS HORMONES

Al-Massadi, O., Fernø, J., Diéguez, C., Nogueiras, R., & Quiñones, M. (2019). Glucagon control on food intake and energy balance. *International Journal of Molecular Sciences, 20*(16), 3905.

Batterham, R. L., Cowley, M. A., Small, C. J., Herzog, H., Cohen, M. A., Dakin, C. L., Wren, A. M., Brynes, A. E., Low, M. J., Ghatei, M. A., Cone, R. D.,

& Bloom, S. R. (2002). Gut hormone PYY (3–36) physiologically inhibits food intake. *Nature* (London), 418(6898), 650–654.

Butler, P. C., Chou, J., Carter, W. B., Wang, Y. N., Bu, B. H., Chang, D., Chang, J. K., & Rizza, R. A. (1990). Effects of meal ingestion on plasma amylin concentration in NIDDM and nondiabetic humans. *Diabetes* (New York, N.Y.), 39(6), 752–756.

Degen, L., Oesch, S., Casanova, M., Graf, S., Ketterer, S., Drewe, J., & Beglinger, C. (2005). Effect of peptide YY3–36 on food intake in humans. *Gastroenterology* (New York, N.Y. 1943), 129(5), 1430–1436.

Karra, E., Chandarana, K., & Batterham, R. L. (2009). The role of peptide YY in appetite regulation and obesity. *Journal of Physiology,* 587(1), 19–25.

Kirkham, T. C., & Harrold, J. A. (2008) The anorectic peptide PYY (3-36) reduces the reinforcing efficacy of food in free-feeding rats. *Journal of Psychopharmacology,* 22(1), 34–41.

Hay, D. L., Chen, S., Lutz, T. A., Parkes, D. G., & Roth, J. D. (2015). Amylin: pharmacology, physiology, and clinical potential. *Pharmacological Reviews,* 67(3), 564–600.

Müller, T. D., Finan, B., Clemmensen, C., DiMarchi, R. D., & Tschöp, M. H. (2017). The new biology and pharmacology of glucagon. *Physiological Reviews,* 97(2), 721–766.

Pocai, A., Carrington, P. E., Liu, F., Miller, C., Tota, L. M., Gaochao Zhou, Xiaoping Zhang, Sountis, M. M., Santoprete, A., Capito, E., Chicchi, G. G., Thornberry, N., Adams, J. R., Bianchi, E., Pessi, A., Marsh, D. J., Sinharoy, R., Wright, M., Eiermann, G., & Jiang, G. (2009). Glucagon-like peptide 1/ glucagon receptor dual agonism reverses obesity in mice. *Diabetes* (New York, N.Y.), 58(10), 2258–2266.

THE CLAIM THAT "LASTING WEIGHT LOSS IS ALMOST IMPOSSIBLE"

Clemmensen, C. & Sjøgren, K. (2020) Forskere jagter årsagen til det vanskelige vedvarende vægttab. Sciencenews/Sciencenews.dk. https:// sciencenews.dk/da/forskere-jagter-aarsagen-til-det-vanskelige -vedvarende-vaegttab.

Jensen, S. L. (2024). He has been researching obesity for more than fifty years. He knows the best possible way to avoid having overweight children. Berlingske Tidende/Berlingske.dk. jttp://www.berlingske.dk/

indland/han-har-forsket-i-fedme-i-mere-end-50-aar-han-ved-hvordan
-du-bedst-muligt?.

Poulsen, A. G. (2021). Ny rapport om forebyggelse af overvægt: vi skal
tænke det hele om. Ugeskriftet/Ugeskriftet.dk. https://ugeskriftet.dk/
nyhed/ny-rapport-om-forebyggelse-af-overvaegt-vi-skal-taenke-det
-hele-om.

Ringgaard, A. (2020). Forskere: Overvægt er sjældent selvforskyldt.
Videnskab DK/Videnskab.dk. https://videnskab.dk/krop-sundhed/
forskere-overvaegt-er-sjaeldent-selvforskyldt/.

Videnskaben bag overvægt/Truth About Weight Global. https://www
.truthaboutweight.global/dk/da/videnskab.html.

BOOKS CONTAINING MORE OF THE SAME

Holst, J. J. (2024). Historien om GLP-1: en forskningshistorisk rejse i
behandlingen af diabetes og svær overvægt. FADL.

Sams, A. (2017). Sandheden om sukker—alt, du skal vide om sukker for at
opnå solid sundhed, undgå inflammation, smid kiloene og styr uden om
livsstilssygdomme. Gyldendal.

Sams, A. (2019). The truth about sugar—avoid inflammation, drop pounds
and steer clear of lifestyle diseases. Gyldendal.

Sams, A., & Faerber, J. (2022). Kålhydrater—Gør kål på overvægt,
insulinresistens og sukkertrang. Gyldendal.

About the author

ANETTE SAMS (1971) is a pharmacist with a PhD from the University of Copenhagen.

After fifteen years as a medical researcher, manager, and director at Novo Nordisk, Anette Sams left her job to enlighten Danes about the body's own biological "health switches" that can help combat obesity, unwanted inflammation, and lifestyle diseases.

Among other things, this has led to four best-selling books, including one that has previously been translated into English, namely *The Truth About Sugar,* published by Gyldendal.

Alongside her work as an author and health advocate, Anette Sams works for a company developing new treatments for serious cardiovascular diseases.